METABOLIC RESET DIET

A Proven Path to Sustainable Weight Loss and Optimal Health: Boost Your Metabolism and Beat Your Body at Its Own Game with a Simple Guide to Delicious Recipes, Meal Plans, and Exercises

Michelle O. Lewis

Copyright © 2023 by **Michelle O. Lewis**

All rights reserved. No part of this book may be used or reproduced in any form whatsoever without written permission except in the case of brief quotations in critical articles or reviews.

Printed in the United States of America.

First Edition: October 2023

TABLE OF CONTENT

Introduction: 1

Understanding Metabolism 1

The Importance of A Metabolic Reset 2

Weight Management: 2
Energy Levels: 2
Hormonal Balance: 2
Improved Nutrient Absorption: 2
Long-Term Health: 3
Gut Health: 3
Mental Well-being: 3
Aging Gracefully: 3
Customization: 3

How This Book Can Help You 4

Unlocking the Power of Your Metabolism: 4
Sustainable Weight Management: 4
Optimal Health and Vitality: 4
Delicious Recipes and Nutritious Meal Plans: 4
Efficient and Sustainable Exercise: 5
Long-Term Success: 5

The Science of Metabolism 6

What Is Metabolism? 6
Definition of Metabolism 6
Metabolism and Homeostasis 7
Factors Influencing Metabolism 7
Metabolism and Health 7

How Metabolism Affects Weight 9

The Metabolic Factors in Weight Management 9
Basal Metabolic Rate (BMR) 9
Total Daily Energy Expenditure (TDEE) 9
Energy Balance 9

Factors Affecting Metabolism and Weight 11

Several factors influence how metabolism impacts weight: 11
Genetics 11
Age 11
Body Composition 11
Diet and Physical Activity 11

Strategies For Weight Management Through Metabolism .. 12

Balanced Diet 12
Physical Activity 12
Adequate Sleep 12
Stress Management 12
Hydration 12

Recent Research and Discoveries 14

Microbiome and Metabolism: 14
Precision Nutrition: 14
Hormonal Regulation: 14
Metabolic Pathways: 14
Metabolism and Aging: 15
Exercise Physiology: 15
Metabolism and Mental Health: 15
Metabolic Phenotyping: 15
Nutritional Supplements and Metabolism: 15
Metabolism and Epigenetics: 15

THE Metabolic Reset Approach 17

What is a Metabolic Reset Diet? 17
Balanced Diet 17
Regular Meals 17
Physical Activity: 17
Adequate Hydration: 17
Adequate Sleep: 17
Stress Management 18
Avoiding Extreme Caloric Restriction 18
Consulting a Healthcare Professional: 18

Goals and Benefits 19

Potential Goals of a Metabolic Reset Diet: 19
Improved Energy Levels: 19
Balanced Blood Sugar: 19
Hormonal Balance: 19
Better Nutrient Utilization: 20

Potential Benefits of a Metabolic Reset Diet: 20
Weight Loss: 20
Increased Energy: 20
Better Blood Sugar Control: 20
Hormonal Balance: 20
Nutrient Optimization: 20
Digestive Health: 20

Who can Benefit from A Metabolic Reset? 22
People with Metabolic Syndrome: 22
Individuals with Insulin Resistance: 22
Overweight or Obese Individuals: 22
Those with Hormonal Imbalances: 23

People with Energy and Fatigue Issues: 23
Those Seeking Improved Athletic Performance: 23
Aging Individuals: 23
Anyone Interested in Overall Health and Well-Being: 23

Common Misconceptions 24

One-Size-Fits-All Approach: 24
Rapid and Dramatic Results: 24
Extreme Caloric Restriction: 24
Supplements and Products: 24
Lack of Individualization: 25
Long-Term Sustainability: 25
Excessive Focus on Specific Foods: 25
Lack of Professional Guidance: 25

Assessing Your Current Metabolism 27

Metabolic Rate Measurements 27

Resting Metabolic Rate (RMR): 27
Harris-Benedict Equation: 27
Bioelectrical Impedance Analysis (BIA): 27
Activity Trackers: 28
Caloric Estimation: 28
Doubly Labeled Water (DLW): 28
Indirect Calorimetry During Exercise 28
Metabolic Cart: 28
Activity Monitors and Wearables: 28

Identifying Metabolic Challenges 30

Unexplained Weight Changes: 30
Fatigue: 30
Changes in Appetite: 30

Blood Sugar Irregularities: 30
High Blood Pressure: 31
High Cholesterol: 31
Digestive Problems: 31
Hormonal Irregularities: 31
Thyroid Dysfunction: 31
Difficulty in Concentration and Memory 31
Skin and Hair Changes: 31
Muscle and Joint Pain 32
Intolerance to Cold or Heat 32

Setting Realistic Goals 33

Define Clear Objectives: 33
Understand Your Starting Point: 33
Consult with a Healthcare Professional: 33
Set Incremental Milestones: 33
Consider Your Resources: 34
Set a Timeframe: 34
Prioritize Balanced Nutrition: 34
Be Mindful of Individual Variation: 34
Monitor and Adjust: 34
Celebrate Small Wins: 34
Stay Informed: 35

Nutritional Foundations 37

Understanding Macronutrients 37

Carbohydrates: 37
Proteins: 37
Fats: 38

Micronutrients for Metabolism 40

1. Vitamin B Complex: 40
2. Vitamin C (Ascorbic Acid): 40
3. Vitamin D: 40
4. Calcium: 40
5. Magnesium: 41
6. Iron: 41
7. Zinc: 41
8. Selenium: 41
9. Copper: 41
10. Chromium: 41
11. Manganese: 42
12. Iodine: 42

Hydration and Metabolism 43

1. Cellular Function: 43
2. Thermoregulation: 43
3. Digestion and Nutrient Transport: 43
4. Blood Circulation: 43
5. Energy Production: 44
6. Kidney Function: 44
7. Detoxification: 44
8. Hormone Regulation: 44
9. Appetite Regulation: 44
10. Weight Management: 44

The Role of Fiber 46

Digestion and Nutrient Absorption: 46
Blood Sugar Regulation: 46
Weight Management: 46
Cholesterol Control: 46

Gut Health: 47
Energy Balance: 47
Thermogenesis: 47
Healthy Body Weight: 47

The Metabolic Reset Diet Plan **48**

Phase 1: Preparing For Reset **48**

1. Goal Setting: 48
2. Assessing Current Habits: 48
3. Consultation: 48
4. Meal Planning: 48
5. Pantry Cleanout: 49
6. Hydration: 49
7. Exercise Plan: 49
8. Stress Management: 49
9. Sleep Hygiene: 49
10. Tracking Progress: 49
11. Meal Prep: 50
12. Support System: 50
13. Educate Yourself: 50
14. Mental Preparedness: 50

Eliminating Harmful Foods **51**

1. Identify Harmful Foods: 51
2. Read Food Labels: 51
3. Reduce Sugary Foods and Drinks: 51
4. Cut Back on Processed Foods: 51
5. Avoid Trans Fats: 52
6. Identify Allergens or Sensitivities: 52
7. Limit Excessive Salt: 52

8.	Minimize Refined Grains:	52
9.	Reduce Red and Processed Meats:	52
10.	Stay Hydrated with Water:	53
11.	Plan Healthy Substitutes:	53
12.	Prepare Meals at Home:	53
13.	Educate Yourself:	53

Meal Prep and Planning 54

1.	Set Clear Goals:	54
2.	Create a Weekly Menu:	54
3.	Balance Macronutrients	54
4.	Control Portion Sizes:	54
5.	Include Fiber:	55
6.	Plan Snacks:	55
7.	Diversify Protein Sources:	55
8.	Prepare Ahead of Time:	55
9.	Use the Right Tools:	55
10.	Label and Date:	55
11.	Refrigerate or Freeze:	56
12.	Plan for Variety:	56
13.	Review and Adjust:	56
14.	Stay Hydrated:	56

Phase 2: Resetting Your Metabolism 57

1.	Follow Your Prepared Meal Plan:	57
2.	Portion Control:	57
3.	Prioritize Nutrient-Dense Foods:	57
4.	Hydration:	57
5.	Regular Meal Timing:	57
6.	Balanced Macronutrients:	58

7.	Reduce Sugar Intake:	58
8.	Manage Stress:	58
9.	Regular Exercise:	58
10.	Quality Sleep:	58
11.	Monitor Progress:	58
12.	Seek Support:	59
13.	Educate Yourself:	59
14.	Stay Mindful:	59
15.	Adapt as Needed:	59

Meal Timing Strategies 60

1.	Regular Meal Schedule:	60
2.	Balanced Breakfast:	60
3.	Frequent, Smaller Meals:	60
4.	Intuitive Eating:	60
5.	Protein Timing:	61
6.	Post-Workout Nutrition:	61
7.	Mid-Morning and Afternoon Snacks:	61
8.	Early Dinner:	61
9.	Avoid Late-Night Snacking:	61
10.	Time-Restricted Eating:	61
11.	Avoid Skipping Meals:	62
12.	Monitor Your Body's Response:	62
13.	Stay Hydrated:	62
14.	Consult a Dietitian:	62

Intermittent Fasting 63

16/8 Method: 63
5:2 Diet: 63
Eat-Stop-Eat: 63

Alternate-Day Fasting 63
The Warrior Diet: 63
OMAD (One Meal a Day): 64

Phase 3: Maintaining A Healthy Metabolism 66

1. Lifestyle Integration: 66
2. Consistency: 66
3. Regular Monitoring: 66
4. Adapt to Changes: 66
5. Support System: 66
6. Education: 67
7. Mindful Eating: 67
8. Hydration: 67
9. Physical Activity: 67
10. Stress Management: 67
11. Quality Sleep: 67
12. Nutrient-Dense Foods: 67
13. Occasional Indulgences: 68
14. Regular Health Checkups: 68
15. Plan for Challenges: 68
16. Long-Term Mindset: 68

Long-Term Nutrition Strategies 69

1. Whole, Unprocessed Foods: 69
2. Portion Control: 69
3. Balanced Macronutrients: 69
4. Fiber-Rich Foods: 69
5. Protein Variety: 69
6. Limit Sugars and Processed Foods: 70
7. Healthy Fats: 70

8.	Regular Meal Timing:	70
9.	Hydration:	70
10.	Mindful Eating:	70
11.	Variety and Moderation	70
12.	Meal Planning:	70
13.	Nutrition Education:	71
14.	Long-Term Goals:	71
15.	Regular Health Checkups:	71
16.	Adapt to Life Changes:	71
17.	Family and Social Support:	71
18.	Seek Professional Guidance:	71

Transitioning Out of Reset Mode 73

Gradual Adjustments: 73
Monitoring: 73
Balance: 73
Consistency: 73
Flexibility: 73
Education: 73
Regular Health Checkups: 74
Support System: 74
Mindful Eating: 74
Stress Management: 74
Quality Sleep: 74
Physical Activity: 74
Variety: 74
Educate Others: 74
Adaptive Goals: 75

Week-By-Week Meal Plans For Each Phase 76

Phase 1: Preparation **76**

Week 1: 76

Phase 2: Reset **78**

Week 2: 78

Phase 3: Maintenance **80**

Week 3: 80

Balanced and Delicious Recipes **83**

BREAKFAST: **83**

1. Greek Yogurt Parfait 83
2. Spinach and Feta Omelette 84
3. Peanut Butter Banana Smoothie 85
4. Veggie and Cheese Breakfast Quesadilla 86
5. Overnight Chia Pudding 87

LUNCH RECIPES: **88**

1. Grilled Chicken and Quinoa Salad 88
2. Chickpea and Avocado Wrap 89
3. Salmon and Quinoa Bowl 90
4. Lentil and Vegetable Stir-Fry 91
5. Caprese Salad with Grilled Chicken 92

DINNER RECIPES: **93**

1. Baked Salmon with Quinoa and Asparagus 93
2. Vegetable Stir-Fry with Tofu 94
3. Grilled Chicken with Sweet Potato and Green Beans 95
4. Lentil and Vegetable Soup 96
5. Quinoa and Black Bean Stuffed Bell Peppers 97

SNACKS RECIPES: **99**

1. Greek Yogurt and Berry Parfait 99
2. Hummus and Veggie Snack Plate 100
3. Almond Butter and Banana Slices 101
4. Trail Mix with Nuts and Dried Fruit 102
5. Cottage Cheese and Pineapple Salsa 103

SMOOTHIE RECIPES: 104

1. Green Spinach and Banana Smoothie 104
2. Berry and Almond Butter Smoothie 105
3. Tropical Mango and Pineapple Smoothie 106
4. Chocolate Protein Smoothie 107
5. Oatmeal and Banana Breakfast Smoothie 108

Portion Control and Calorie Management 109

Portion Control: 109

- Use Measuring Tools: 109
- Learn Visual Cues: 109
- Use Smaller Plates: 109
- Divide Your Plate: 109
- Avoid Eating Directly from Packages: 110
- Listen to Hunger Cues: 110

Calorie Management: 110

- Determine Your Caloric Needs: 110
- Track Your Intake: 110
- Read Nutrition Labels: 110
- Understand Caloric Density: 111
- Monitor Beverages: 111
- Practice Moderation: 111
- Plan Balanced Meals: 111
- Stay Active: 111

Exercise and Metabolism 112
The Role of Exercise in Metabolic Reset 112

1. Caloric Expenditure: 112
2. Muscle Maintenance and Growth: 112
3. Metabolic Rate: 112
4. Hormone Regulation: 112
5. Appetite Control: 113
6. Improved Energy Levels: 113
7. Cardiovascular Health: 113
8. Stress Reduction: 113
9. Metabolic Flexibility: 113

Metabolism-Boosting Workouts 115

Strength Training: 115
High-Intensity Interval Training (HIIT): 115
Circuit Training: 115
Cardiovascular Exercise: 115
Compound Movements: 116
Metabolic Conditioning Workouts: 116
Tabata Workouts: 116
Functional Fitness: 116
Plyometrics: 116
Core and Stability Training: 116
Yoga and Pilates: 117

Combining Diet and Exercise For Optimal Results 118

1. Set Clear Goals: 118
2. Balanced Diet: 118
3. Macronutrient Balance: 118
4. Meal Timing: 118

5. Stay Hydrated: 119
6. Portion Control: 119
7. Quality Over Quantity: 119
8. Consistency: 119
9. Monitor Progress: 119
10. Adapt and Adjust: 119
11. Seek Professional Guidance: 119
12. Rest and Recovery: 120
13. Mindful Eating: 120
14. Stress Management: 120

Tracking and Monitoring Progress 121

Setting Milestones 121

1. Define Specific Goals: 121
2. Break Goals into Smaller Steps: 121
3. Make Them SMART: 121
4. Quantify Your Progress: 121
5. Create a Timeline: 122
6. Celebrate Achievements: 122
7. Adjust and Reflect: 122
8. Stay Accountable: 122
9. Document Your Journey: 123
10. Embrace Setbacks as Learning Opportunities: 123
11. Adjust for Lifestyle Changes: 123
12. Reflect on Non-Scale Wins: 123
13. Seek Professional Guidance: 123

Keeping A Food Diary 124

1. Choose a Format: 124
2. Be Consistent: 124

3. Record Portion Sizes: 124

4. Note the Time: 124

5. Describe Food Preparation: 125

6. Include Snacks and Drinks: 125

7. Be Honest: 125

8. Track Emotions and Circumstances: 125

9. Analyze Your Data: 125

10. Set Specific Goals: 126

11. Seek Professional Guidance: 126

12. Use It as a Learning Tool: 126

13. Plan Ahead: 126

14. Monitor Progress: 126

15. Adapt and Make Changes: 126

Using Technology and Apps 128

1. Food Tracking Apps: 128

2. Calorie and Macronutrient Calculators: 128

3. Meal Planning Apps: 128

4. Fitness Trackers: 128

5. Health Apps: 129

6. Recipe Apps: 129

7. Nutrition Education Apps: 129

8. Fitness and Workout Apps: 129

9. Hydration Apps: 129

10. Mindfulness and Stress Reduction Apps: 130

11. Goal-Setting Apps: 130

12. Social and Support Apps: 130

13. Telehealth Apps: 130

14. Biometric and Health Monitoring Devices: 130

15. Data Analysis and Visualization Tools: 131

16. Wearable Nutrition Sensors: 131
17. Personalized Diet Apps: 131

Overcoming Plateaus and Challenges 132

Common Roadblocks 132

1. Lack of Motivation: 132
2. Unrealistic Expectations: 132
3. Plateaus: 132
4. Emotional Eating: 133
5. Social Pressure: 133
6. Lack of Time: 133
7. Boredom: 133
8. Overwhelm: 133
9. Lack of Support: 134
10. Medical Issues: 134
11. Inconsistent Self-Care: 134
12. Self-Criticism: 134
13. Financial Constraints: 135
14. Sustainability: 135

Strategies for Breaking Plateaus 136

1. Change Your Workout Routine: 136
2. Increase Intensity: 136
3. Cross-Training: 136
4. Track Your Progress: 136
5. Reevaluate Your Diet: 137
6. Add More Protein: 137
7. Manage Stress: 137
8. Prioritize Sleep: 137
9. Stay Hydrated: 137

10. Refeed Days: 138
11. Be Patient: 138
12. Consult a Professional: 138
13. Mental Resilience: 138
14. Reassess Goals: 138
15. Seek Social Support: 139
16. Listen to Your Body: 139

Dealing With Cravings and Emotional Eating **140**

1. Self-Awareness: 140
2. Practice Mindfulness: 140
3. Keep a Food Diary: 140
4. Find Alternatives: 140
5. Stay Hydrated: 141
6. Balanced Meals: 141
7. Plan Your Meals: 141
8. Avoid Extreme Diets: 141
9. Stress Management: 141
10. Emotional Support: 141
11. Avoid Triggers: 142
12. Delay and Distract: 142
13. Practice Portion Control: 142
14. Find Healthy Outlets: 142
15. Seek Professional Help: 142
16. Be Kind to Yourself: 143

Success Stories and Case Studies **144**

Real-Life Testimonials **144**

Testimonial 1: Naomi's Metabolic Reset Journey 144
Testimonial 2: John's Metabolic Reset Success 145

Testimonial 3: Maria's Transformation Story 147

Testimonial 4: Mark's Health Rebirth 148

Analyzing Successful Transformations 151

1. Clear Goals: 151
2. Education and Knowledge: 151
3. Balanced Diet: 151
4. Portion Control: 151
5. Regular Exercise: 152
6. Consistency: 152
7. Accountability: 152
8. Stress Management: 152
9. Adaptable Approach: 152
10. Patience: 153
11. Regular Monitoring: 153
12. Celebrating Milestones: 153
13. Professional Guidance: 153
14. Lifestyle Integration: 153

Inspiration for Your Journey 155

Maintaining a Healthy Metabolism for Life 158

Post-Metabolic Reset Guidelines 158

1. Maintain Your New Habits: 158
2. Regular Check-Ins: 158
3. Balanced Diet: 158
4. Mindful Eating: 158
5. Regular Exercise: 159
6. Stay Hydrated: 159
7. Manage Stress: 159
8. Sleep: 159

9. Celebrate Success: 159
10. Be Adaptable: 159
11. Support System: 160
12. Learn Continuously: 160
13. Periodic Assessments: 160
14. Set New Goals: 160
15. Long-Term Perspective: 160
16. Help Others: 160

Incorporating Variety into Your Diet **162**

1. Explore Different Food Groups: 162
2. Seasonal Eating: 162
3. Try New Recipes: 162
4. Mix Protein Sources: 162
5. Colorful Plates: 163
6. Whole Grains Variety: 163
7. Experiment with Spices and Herbs: 163
8. Meal Planning: 163
9. Seasonal Fruits and Vegetables: 163
10. Food Swaps: 163
11. Breakfast Variations: 164
12. Snack Smart: 164
13. Cultural Exploration: 164
14. Listen to Cravings: 164
15. Regularly Update Your Grocery List: 164
16. Share Meals: 164

Beyond Weight Loss **166**

Improving Energy Levels **166**

Balanced Diet: 166

Regular Meals: 166
Stay Hydrated: 166
Control Portion Sizes: 166
Complex Carbohydrates: 167
Protein Intake: 167
Healthy Fats: 167
Limit Added Sugars: 167
Fiber-Rich Foods: 167
Balanced Snacks: 167
Regular Exercise: 168
Manage Stress: 168
Adequate Sleep: 168
Limit Caffeine and Alcohol: 168
Regular Mealtimes: 168
Stay Active: 168
Hydrotherapy: 169
Breathe Deeply: 169
Set Realistic Goals: 169
Stay Positive: 169

Supporting Overall Wellness 170

1. Balanced Nutrition: 170
2. Regular Exercise: 170
3. Hydration: 170
4. Quality Sleep: 170
5. Stress Management: 171
6. Mental Health Support: 171
7. Social Connections: 171
8. Purpose and Meaning: 171
9. Time Management: 171

10. Regular Check-Ups: 171
11. Self-Care: 172
12. Holistic Wellness: 172
13. Goal Setting: 172
14. Environmental Wellness: 172
15. Spiritual Wellness: 172
16. Financial Wellness: 172
17. Lifelong Learning: 173
18. Gratitude and Positivity: 173
19. Giving Back: 173
20. Balance and Adaptability: 173

Conclusion 174

Your Future with A Revitalized Metabolism 174

1. Lifelong Well-Being: 174
2. Preventative Health: 174
3. Improved Energy: 174
4. Mental Clarity: 174
5. Emotional Well-Being: 175
6. Physical Fitness: 175
7. Longevity: 175
8. Positive Habits: 175
9. Personal Growth: 175
10. Inspirational Impact: 175

INTRODUCTION:

UNDERSTANDING METABOLISM

Metabolism is a fundamental and intricate biological process that occurs within all living organisms, including humans. It encompasses a series of chemical reactions that enable an organism to acquire, transform, store, and utilize energy derived from the nutrients in its environment. This complex network of reactions is essential for maintaining life, as it supports various functions, such as growth, reproduction, and the regulation of bodily processes.

Metabolism can be broadly categorized into two main components: catabolism and anabolism. Catabolism involves the breakdown of complex molecules into simpler ones, releasing energy in the process. Conversely, anabolism entails the synthesis of complex molecules from simpler ones, consuming energy in the process. Together, these processes are tightly regulated and orchestrated to maintain the delicate balance of energy production and utilization in an organism.

Understanding metabolism is critical not only for grasping the fundamentals of biology but also for various aspects of human health and medicine. Dysregulation of metabolism can lead to various health issues, including obesity, diabetes, and metabolic disorders. Therefore, it is essential to explore the intricate mechanisms of metabolism, including its key components, factors influencing it, and its role in maintaining overall well-being. This understanding allows for the development of strategies to manage and improve metabolic health, impacting the quality of life for individuals and populations alike.

THE IMPORTANCE OF A METABOLIC RESET

A metabolic reset, sometimes referred to as metabolic resetting, is the concept of making intentional changes to your diet, exercise, and lifestyle in order to optimize your metabolism. This process is gaining attention in the field of health and wellness for several important reasons:

Weight Management: A properly functioning metabolism is crucial for maintaining a healthy weight. When your metabolism is out of balance, it can be difficult to lose weight or prevent weight gain. A metabolic reset can help kickstart weight loss by improving your body's ability to burn calories efficiently.

Energy Levels: Metabolism plays a key role in providing your body with the energy it needs to perform everyday activities. A well-balanced metabolism can help boost energy levels, making you feel more alert and active throughout the day.

Hormonal Balance: Metabolism is intricately connected to hormone regulation. A metabolic reset can help balance hormones like insulin and leptin, which are critical for appetite control and fat storage. This balance can have a positive impact on conditions like diabetes and metabolic syndrome.

Improved Nutrient Absorption: An optimized metabolism can enhance your body's ability to absorb and utilize nutrients from the food you eat. This is essential for overall health and can prevent deficiencies in essential vitamins and minerals.

Long-Term Health: A metabolic reset can have a lasting impact on your overall health. By promoting a healthy metabolism, you reduce the risk of developing chronic diseases like type 2 diabetes, cardiovascular disease, and certain cancers.

Gut Health: The gut microbiome, which plays a significant role in metabolism, can be positively influenced by dietary and lifestyle changes. A metabolic reset often includes improvements in gut health, which can have far-reaching benefits.

Mental Well-being: A well-functioning metabolism can also have a positive impact on mental health. Stable blood sugar levels, for example, can reduce mood swings and irritability.

Aging Gracefully: As we age, our metabolism naturally slows down. A metabolic reset can help mitigate some of the effects of aging on metabolism and overall health.

Customization: A metabolic reset plan can be tailored to an individual's unique needs and goals. It can be adapted for those looking to lose weight, build muscle, or simply improve overall well-being.

To achieve a metabolic reset, it is essential to consider factors such as diet, exercise, stress management, sleep, and hydration. Consulting with a healthcare professional or a registered dietitian can be particularly helpful in designing a personalized plan that addresses your specific metabolic needs and goals. In summary, a metabolic reset is an important strategy for improving health, managing weight, and promoting overall well-being.

HOW THIS BOOK CAN HELP YOU

This book is your comprehensive guide to achieving a significant transformation in your health and wellness. Here's how it can empower you to achieve your goals:

Unlocking the Power of Your Metabolism: We will demystify the complex world of metabolism and provide you with a clear understanding of how it affects your weight, energy levels, and overall health. Armed with this knowledge, you'll be better equipped to make informed decisions about your diet and lifestyle.

Sustainable Weight Management: This book offers a proven approach to sustainable weight loss and maintenance. You'll learn to shed unwanted pounds without resorting to crash diets or extreme measures. Our strategies are built on scientific findings and designed to help you reach your weight management goals while enjoying a balanced and satisfying diet.

Optimal Health and Vitality: Your metabolism plays a crucial role in your overall well-being. By following the guidance in this book, you'll not only achieve your weight-related objectives but also experience a surge in energy levels, improved vitality, and enhanced health. We provide you with the tools to optimize your metabolism and promote lifelong wellness.

Delicious Recipes and Nutritious Meal Plans: Practicality is at the core of our approach. You'll gain access to delectable recipes and customized meal plans that make your metabolic reset journey enjoyable and easy to follow. These recipes are designed to support your health and weight goals while satisfying your taste buds.

Efficient and Sustainable Exercise: Our book includes straightforward workout strategies that complement your metabolic reset. You'll discover how to incorporate exercise into your routine without the need for extreme training regimens. These fitness plans are tailored to maximize the benefits of your metabolic reset journey.

Long-Term Success: We're not interested in providing short-lived solutions. This book equips you with the knowledge and tools to maintain your progress well beyond the initial phase of your metabolic reset. It's a lasting transformation that's within your reach.

By embracing the insights and strategies presented in this book, you can take control of your metabolism, redefine your health and wellness, and embark on a path to a revitalized, healthier you. This book is your key to understanding, embracing, and harnessing the incredible potential of your metabolism for a lifetime of well-being.

CHAPTER ONE
THE SCIENCE OF METABOLISM

What Is Metabolism?

Metabolism is one of the most fundamental processes in biology, serving as the engine that powers life itself. It encompasses a complex series of chemical reactions within an organism, enabling it to acquire, convert, store, and utilize energy derived from the nutrients it obtains from its environment. Understanding the basics of metabolism is essential for comprehending how living organisms function and how they sustain life.

Definition of Metabolism

Metabolism, in its simplest terms, can be defined as the sum of all chemical reactions that occur within an organism. These reactions are responsible for maintaining various essential functions, including:

1. Anabolism: This aspect of metabolism involves the synthesis of complex molecules from simpler ones. It consumes energy and is responsible for processes like building proteins, DNA, and other cell components.

2. Catabolism: Catabolism is the opposite of anabolism, involving the breakdown of complex molecules into simpler ones. This process releases energy, which is then used to power various cellular functions.

1.1.2 Energy Production and Consumption

Central to metabolism is the concept of energy production and consumption. Organisms need energy to perform tasks ranging from basic cellular functions to complex activities like walking, thinking, and reproducing. This energy primarily comes from the food an organism consumes. The process by which cells extract energy from nutrients is called cellular respiration, which involves the breakdown of glucose and other molecules to produce a molecule called adenosine triphosphate (ATP). ATP serves as the primary energy currency of cells.

Metabolism and Homeostasis

Metabolism plays a critical role in maintaining the internal environment of an organism, a state known as homeostasis. It regulates factors like body temperature, blood sugar levels, and hormone balance. When these processes are disrupted, it can lead to health issues and diseases.

Factors Influencing Metabolism

Metabolism varies among individuals, influenced by factors such as genetics, age, gender, and body composition. Some people naturally have faster metabolisms, while others have slower ones. Understanding these factors is vital for tailoring strategies to optimize metabolism and overall health.

Metabolism and Health

Metabolism is closely tied to overall health. Dysregulation of metabolism can lead to various health problems, including obesity, diabetes, and metabolic disorders. Thus, gaining a deeper understanding of metabolism is essential for managing and improving health and well-being.

In the subsequent chapters of this book, we will delve deeper into the intricacies of metabolism, exploring the specific biochemical pathways, hormonal regulations, and lifestyle factors that influence this critical biological process. This knowledge will empower you to make informed choices about your diet, exercise, and overall lifestyle to promote a healthier metabolism and a more fulfilling life.

HOW METABOLISM AFFECTS WEIGHT

The Metabolic Factors in Weight Management

Metabolism plays a pivotal role in determining an individual's body weight and body composition. Understanding the intricate relationship between metabolism and weight is essential for anyone striving to achieve or maintain a healthy body weight.

Basal Metabolic Rate (BMR)

One of the key ways in which metabolism affects weight is through the Basal Metabolic Rate (BMR). BMR represents the energy your body expends at rest to maintain essential functions such as breathing, circulating blood, and cell repair. A higher BMR means your body burns more calories at rest, making it easier to maintain a healthy weight.

Total Daily Energy Expenditure (TDEE)

TDEE is the total number of calories your body burns in a day, encompassing not only BMR but also calories burned through physical activity and the thermic effect of food (calories burned during digestion). Variations in BMR and physical activity levels among individuals can result in differences in TDEE.

Energy Balance

Weight management is fundamentally determined by energy balance, which is the relationship between the calories you consume (through food and beverages) and the calories you expend (through metabolism and physical activity).

Caloric Surplus: If you consume more calories than your body needs (positive energy balance), the excess calories are stored as fat, leading to weight gain.

Caloric Deficit: If you consume fewer calories than your body needs (negative energy balance), your body uses stored energy reserves (fat) to meet its energy demands, resulting in weight loss.

FACTORS AFFECTING METABOLISM AND WEIGHT

Several factors influence how metabolism impacts weight:

Genetics

Genetics can influence an individual's BMR, fat storage tendencies, and even their response to certain diets. Some people may inherit genes that predispose them to a faster or slower metabolism, which can affect their propensity to gain or lose weight.

Age

Metabolism tends to naturally slow down with age. This is largely due to decreases in muscle mass and hormonal changes. As you age, it becomes more challenging to maintain a healthy weight without making dietary and lifestyle adjustments.

Body Composition

Muscle tissue burns more calories at rest than fat tissue. Individuals with a higher proportion of muscle relative to fat tend to have a higher BMR, making it easier to manage their weight.

Diet and Physical Activity

Diet and physical activity choices have a direct impact on metabolism and, consequently, weight. Eating a diet rich in nutrient-dense foods and engaging in regular physical activity can boost your metabolism, while a sedentary lifestyle and unhealthy eating habits can slow it down.

STRATEGIES FOR WEIGHT MANAGEMENT THROUGH METABOLISM

Managing weight through metabolism involves a combination of approaches:

Balanced Diet

Consume a balanced diet that provides the necessary nutrients without excessive calories. This ensures that your metabolism has the fuel it needs to function optimally.

Physical Activity

Engage in regular physical activity, including both cardiovascular exercises and strength training, to increase muscle mass and boost metabolism.

Adequate Sleep

Prioritize getting enough quality sleep, as sleep deprivation can disrupt hormone regulation and lead to weight gain.

Stress Management

Chronic stress can negatively impact metabolism. Utilize stress-reduction techniques such as meditation and relaxation exercises.

Hydration

Staying well-hydrated is essential for metabolism to function efficiently.

In the following chapters, we will delve deeper into the role of nutrition, exercise, and other lifestyle factors in influencing metabolism and weight. By understanding these factors and applying evidence-based strategies, you can harness the power of metabolism to achieve and maintain a healthy weight.

RECENT RESEARCH AND DISCOVERIES

Metabolic Health and Disease: Ongoing research explores the connection between metabolism and various health conditions, including obesity, type 2 diabetes, and metabolic syndrome. New discoveries in this area may lead to novel treatments and interventions.

Microbiome and Metabolism: The gut microbiome's role in metabolism and overall health has been a growing area of interest. Research may uncover how specific microbial communities influence metabolic processes.

Precision Nutrition: Tailoring diets to an individual's unique genetic and metabolic profile is an emerging field. Recent studies may provide insights into personalized nutrition and its effects on metabolism.

Hormonal Regulation: Advances in our understanding of hormones such as insulin, leptin, and ghrelin and their roles in metabolism can have significant implications for diabetes management and weight control.

Metabolic Pathways: Ongoing research seeks to unravel the intricate biochemical pathways involved in metabolism. Discoveries in this area could lead to a deeper understanding of metabolic processes and potential therapeutic targets.

Metabolism and Aging: As the population ages, research into the effects of aging on metabolism and strategies to mitigate its impact continues to be a focus of scientific inquiry.

Exercise Physiology: New findings in exercise science and how physical activity influences metabolism can inform more effective exercise regimens for weight management and overall health.

Metabolism and Mental Health: Research on the connection between metabolic health and mental well-being, including conditions like depression and anxiety, is an evolving area.

Metabolic Phenotyping: Advances in technology, including metabolomics, allow for detailed profiling of an individual's metabolic state. Recent research may have uncovered new biomarkers and patterns associated with metabolic health.

Nutritional Supplements and Metabolism: Studies on the effects of various dietary supplements and their impact on metabolic health may yield valuable insights.

Metabolism and Epigenetics: Research into how environmental factors can influence gene expression and metabolism is an exciting frontier in understanding the interplay between nature and nurture in metabolic health.

Remember that scientific research is an ongoing process and new discoveries are made regularly. To access the most recent research and discoveries, consider visiting academic journals, university websites, and reputable news sources specializing in science and health.

CHAPTER TWO

THE METABOLIC RESET APPROACH

WHAT IS A METABOLIC RESET DIET?

The concept of a "metabolic reset" often implies the idea of improving or resetting one's metabolism, In general, approaches to reset metabolism would typically involve changes in diet, physical activity, and lifestyle to promote a healthier metabolic state. These changes may include:

Balanced Diet: Eating a well-balanced diet that includes a variety of nutrient-dense foods such as lean proteins, whole grains, fruits, vegetables, and healthy fats.

Regular Meals: Eating regular meals and snacks throughout the day to prevent extreme fluctuations in blood sugar and energy levels.

Physical Activity: Engaging in regular physical activity, including both cardiovascular exercise and strength training, to help maintain and build muscle mass.

Adequate Hydration: Staying well-hydrated to support various metabolic processes.

Adequate Sleep: Getting enough quality sleep, as sleep plays a significant role in metabolic regulation.

Stress Management: Managing stress through relaxation techniques, meditation, or other stress-reduction methods, as chronic stress can impact metabolism.

Avoiding Extreme Caloric Restriction: Avoid crash diets or extreme caloric restrictions, as they can slow down metabolism over time.

Consulting a Healthcare Professional: If you have specific health concerns or goals related to your metabolism, it's advisable to consult a registered dietitian or healthcare professional who can provide personalized guidance and recommendations based on your individual needs and circumstances.

The key to a healthy metabolism and overall well-being is adopting sustainable and balanced lifestyle changes. Any diet or program that claims to reset your metabolism should be approached with caution and ideally discussed with a healthcare professional to ensure it aligns with your health goals and is based on sound scientific principles.

GOALS AND BENEFITS

The term "metabolic reset diet" is not a widely recognized in the field of nutrition or medicine. However, if we were to speculate on the potential goals and benefits that someone might associate with such a diet based on general principles of health and nutrition, they could include:

POTENTIAL GOALS OF A METABOLIC RESET DIET:

Weight Management: Many people might consider a metabolic reset diet with the goal of losing weight or maintaining a healthy weight. A balanced metabolism is essential for efficient calorie burning and weight control.

Improved Energy Levels: Resetting one's metabolism could aim to improve energy levels by optimizing how the body uses nutrients for energy production.

Balanced Blood Sugar: Some individuals may be interested in stabilizing blood sugar levels, which can be achieved through dietary modifications that support insulin sensitivity and glucose regulation.

Hormonal Balance: Balancing metabolic processes could lead to improved hormonal regulation, which can impact various aspects of health, including mood, fertility, and more.

Better Nutrient Utilization: The goal might be to ensure the body effectively utilizes the nutrients from the diet, thereby promoting overall health and well-being.

POTENTIAL BENEFITS OF A METABOLIC RESET DIET:

Weight Loss: If executed correctly, a metabolic reset diet could lead to weight loss or weight maintenance, which can have numerous health benefits, including reduced risk of chronic diseases.

Increased Energy: A balanced metabolism can result in increased energy levels, making it easier to engage in physical activity and daily tasks.

Better Blood Sugar Control: Improved blood sugar control can reduce the risk of insulin resistance and type 2 diabetes.

Hormonal Balance: A metabolic reset diet might help improve hormonal balance, potentially benefiting individuals with hormonal issues such as polycystic ovary syndrome (PCOS) or thyroid disorders.

Nutrient Optimization: By optimizing nutrient utilization, the diet could support overall health, immune function, and general well-being.

Digestive Health: Dietary changes that promote a metabolic reset may also support digestive health by encouraging the consumption of fiber-rich foods and other gut-friendly choices.

It's important to emphasize that the term "metabolic reset diet" is not well-defined, and the specific goals and benefits can vary depending on the approach one takes. Additionally, the effectiveness and safety of such diets would depend on the specific dietary guidelines and recommendations used, which may not have scientific consensus or validation. Before embarking on any diet, especially one with unconventional claims, it's advisable to consult with a healthcare professional or registered dietitian to ensure that it aligns with your individual health goals and needs.

WHO CAN BENEFIT FROM A METABOLIC RESET?

Considering the broader idea of improving metabolic health and efficiency, there are specific groups of people who might benefit from dietary and lifestyle changes aimed at optimizing their metabolism. Potential candidates who could benefit from efforts to improve metabolic health include:

People with Metabolic Syndrome: Metabolic syndrome is a cluster of conditions, including high blood pressure, high blood sugar, excess abdominal fat, and abnormal cholesterol levels. Individuals with metabolic syndrome may benefit from dietary changes to improve these risk factors and reduce their risk of heart disease and type 2 diabetes.

Individuals with Insulin Resistance: Insulin resistance is a condition in which the body's cells do not respond effectively to insulin, leading to elevated blood sugar levels. Dietary changes can help improve insulin sensitivity and blood sugar control.

Overweight or Obese Individuals: People who are overweight or obese may benefit from a metabolic reset focused on weight management, which can reduce the risk of obesity-related health conditions such as heart disease, type 2 diabetes, and certain types of cancer.

Those with Hormonal Imbalances: Conditions such as polycystic ovary syndrome (PCOS) and thyroid disorders can affect hormonal balance and metabolism. Dietary modifications can potentially help manage symptoms and improve hormonal regulation.

People with Energy and Fatigue Issues: Individuals who experience chronic fatigue or low energy levels may benefit from dietary and lifestyle changes that aim to optimize nutrient intake and energy production within the body.

Those Seeking Improved Athletic Performance: Athletes or individuals engaged in regular physical activity may be interested in optimizing their metabolism to improve energy levels, endurance, and performance.

Aging Individuals: Metabolism tends to slow down with age, and older adults may be interested in dietary strategies that help maintain muscle mass, energy levels, and overall health as they age.

Anyone Interested in Overall Health and Well-Being: In general, many people can benefit from adopting a balanced and health-conscious approach to their diet and lifestyle. Such an approach can support overall health, reduce the risk of chronic diseases, and promote general well-being.

It's important to note that while there is no standardized "metabolic reset" diet, the principles of balanced nutrition, regular physical activity, and a healthy lifestyle apply to most individuals looking to improve their metabolic health. Before making significant dietary changes or embarking on any diet plan, it's advisable to consult with a healthcare professional or registered dietitian to ensure that the approach aligns with your specific health goals and needs.

COMMON MISCONCEPTIONS

There are several common misconceptions or misunderstandings associated with this term. Here are some of the common misconceptions:

One-Size-Fits-All Approach: One of the most significant misconceptions is the idea that there is a single, universal "metabolic reset" diet that works for everyone. In reality, individual dietary needs and goals vary greatly, and there is no one-size-fits-all approach to nutrition.

Rapid and Dramatic Results: Some people may mistakenly believe that a metabolic reset diet can lead to rapid and dramatic results, such as extremely fast weight loss or a sudden increase in energy levels. Sustainable changes in metabolism typically occur gradually and are influenced by various factors, including genetics and lifestyle.

Extreme Caloric Restriction: Some diets claiming to be "metabolic resets" may involve extreme caloric restriction or severely limiting specific nutrients, which can be detrimental to overall health and lead to a slowed metabolism over time.

Supplements and Products: There may be misconceptions that specific supplements, products, or proprietary foods are essential for a metabolic reset diet. It's important to approach such claims with caution and verify their scientific validity.

Lack of Individualization: Metabolism varies from person to person, and any dietary approach should be individualized to address specific needs and goals. A one-size-fits-all approach may not be effective or sustainable.

Long-Term Sustainability: Some diets labeled as metabolic resets may not be sustainable in the long term. A diet that is overly restrictive or unbalanced may be challenging to maintain, which can lead to yo-yo dieting and weight regain.

Excessive Focus on Specific Foods: People may believe that a particular food or food group is the key to a metabolic reset, neglecting the importance of overall dietary patterns and a balanced intake of nutrients.

Lack of Professional Guidance: Without guidance from a healthcare professional or registered dietitian, individuals may attempt a metabolic reset diet without proper evaluation and understanding of their unique needs and circumstances.

It's important to be critical of any diet or nutrition plan that lacks a solid scientific foundation or makes grand claims without proper evidence. Instead, focus on making sustainable, balanced, and evidence-based dietary and lifestyle choices that support your individual health goals and overall well-being. Consulting with a healthcare professional or registered dietitian can provide personalized guidance based on your specific needs and circumstances.

CHAPTER THREE

ASSESSING YOUR CURRENT METABOLISM

METABOLIC RATE MEASUREMENTS

Measuring metabolic rate is a way to quantify how much energy your body uses at rest or during various activities. This information can be valuable for understanding your energy needs, managing weight, and optimizing health and fitness. Several methods are used to measure metabolic rate:

Resting Metabolic Rate (RMR):

Indirect Calorimetry: This is considered the gold standard for measuring RMR. It involves analyzing the gases you exhale (particularly oxygen consumption and carbon dioxide production) to estimate your energy expenditure. This is typically done in a clinical setting using specialized equipment.

Harris-Benedict Equation: This is a formula that estimates RMR based on your age, gender, weight, and height. While it provides a rough estimate, it may not be as accurate as indirect calorimetry.

Bioelectrical Impedance Analysis (BIA): Some BIA devices claim to estimate RMR as part of their measurements. BIA measures electrical impedance through the body to estimate body composition, which can then be used to estimate RMR.

Total Daily Energy Expenditure (TDEE): TDEE includes your RMR plus the energy expended through physical activity and the thermic effect of food (calories burned during digestion). To measure TDEE, people often use various methods:

Activity Trackers: Wearable devices can estimate calorie expenditure based on factors like heart rate, activity level, and body movement.

Caloric Estimation: Apps and online calculators can provide rough estimates of TDEE based on your activity level and dietary intake.

Doubly Labeled Water (DLW): This is a highly accurate method for estimating TDEE over an extended period. It involves consuming water with isotopes and measuring the elimination rate of these isotopes from the body over several days.

Indirect Calorimetry During Exercise: This method measures the energy expenditure during physical activity by analyzing the gases you exhale. It is particularly useful for athletes and individuals seeking precise data on energy expenditure during specific exercises.

Metabolic Cart: This is a portable version of the equipment used in clinical indirect calorimetry. It measures the gases you breathe out to estimate energy expenditure during exercise, making it useful for research and athletic performance assessments.

Activity Monitors and Wearables: Devices like heart rate monitors, fitness trackers, and smartwatches often estimate energy expenditure during exercise based on factors like heart rate, activity type, and duration.

It's important to note that the accuracy of these methods can vary. The best method for measuring metabolic rate depends on the specific goals and circumstances. If you are interested in getting precise measurements for medical, research, or athletic purposes, it's advisable to consult with healthcare professionals or researchers who have access to specialized equipment. For most individuals, estimating metabolic rate using equations and activity trackers can provide a reasonably accurate picture of energy needs for daily activities and goal-setting.

IDENTIFYING METABOLIC CHALLENGES

Identifying metabolic challenges typically involves recognizing signs and symptoms that may indicate underlying metabolic issues. Metabolism is a complex process, and imbalances can lead to various health problems. If you suspect you have metabolic challenges, it's essential to consult with a healthcare professional for a proper diagnosis and guidance. Here are some common signs and symptoms that might suggest metabolic challenges:

Unexplained Weight Changes: Sudden and unexplained weight gain or loss, especially when not related to changes in diet or activity, could indicate a metabolic issue. This includes conditions like hypothyroidism, hyperthyroidism, and insulin resistance.

Fatigue: Chronic fatigue that is not relieved by rest can be a sign of metabolic problems. Conditions like adrenal fatigue, chronic fatigue syndrome, and metabolic syndrome may lead to persistent tiredness.

Changes in Appetite: Significant changes in appetite, such as excessive hunger or loss of appetite, may be linked to metabolic issues, diabetes, or thyroid dysfunction.

Blood Sugar Irregularities: Frequent or severe fluctuations in blood sugar levels, as seen in hypoglycemia or hyperglycemia, may indicate metabolic challenges, particularly diabetes or impaired glucose metabolism.

High Blood Pressure: Hypertension (high blood pressure) can be related to metabolic disorders, such as metabolic syndrome or insulin resistance.

High Cholesterol: Elevated levels of LDL cholesterol, triglycerides, and low levels of HDL cholesterol may be associated with metabolic problems, particularly those linked to heart health.

Digestive Problems: Gastrointestinal issues like irritable bowel syndrome (IBS) or chronic constipation may be influenced by metabolic imbalances.

Hormonal Irregularities: Disorders related to the endocrine system, such as polycystic ovary syndrome (PCOS), irregular menstruation, or hormonal imbalances, can be signs of metabolic challenges.

Thyroid Dysfunction: Symptoms of an underactive thyroid (hypothyroidism), such as fatigue, weight gain, cold intolerance, and hair loss, can indicate a metabolic issue.

Difficulty in Concentration and Memory: Brain fog, poor concentration, and memory issues can sometimes be linked to metabolic disorders.

Skin and Hair Changes: Changes in skin texture, hair loss, and the development of skin conditions like acanthosis nigricans (dark, velvety patches of skin) may be associated with metabolic issues.

Muscle and Joint Pain: Unexplained muscle and joint pain can be linked to metabolic disorders like fibromyalgia or other autoimmune conditions.

Intolerance to Cold or Heat: An inability to tolerate temperature extremes can be associated with thyroid issues or other metabolic problems.

If you're experiencing one or more of these symptoms or have concerns about your metabolic health, it's crucial to consult a healthcare professional. They can conduct appropriate tests and assessments to diagnose any underlying metabolic issues and develop a personalized treatment plan to address your specific needs. Early detection and intervention can help manage or mitigate metabolic challenges and promote overall well-being.

SETTING REALISTIC GOALS

If you're considering dietary changes to improve your metabolic health, here's how you can set realistic goals:

Define Clear Objectives: Begin by clearly defining what you want to achieve with your metabolic reset diet. For example, your goal might be to stabilize blood sugar levels, improve energy levels, manage weight, or optimize hormonal balance. The more specific your goal, the easier it is to work toward.

Understand Your Starting Point: Assess your current metabolic health and identify areas that need improvement. This can include factors like body weight, blood sugar levels, cholesterol, energy levels, and overall well-being.

Consult with a Healthcare Professional: It's crucial to consult with a healthcare professional or a registered dietitian who can help you understand your individual metabolic needs and challenges. They can provide guidance based on your current health status, dietary habits, and lifestyle.

Set Incremental Milestones: Instead of aiming for an immediate and dramatic metabolic reset, break your goal into smaller, achievable milestones. For instance, you might aim to reduce your daily sugar intake, increase your daily fiber intake, or engage in regular physical activity.

Consider Your Resources: Be realistic about the resources at your disposal, including time, knowledge, and budget. Setting goals that require resources you don't have can lead to frustration and failure.

Set a Timeframe: Establish a realistic timeframe for achieving your metabolic health goals. Understand that metabolic changes may take time and that immediate results are not always feasible.

Prioritize Balanced Nutrition: Ensure that your dietary goals are balanced and based on sound nutritional principles. Avoid extreme diets or restrictions that are difficult to maintain in the long term.

Be Mindful of Individual Variation: Metabolism varies from person to person, and what works for one individual may not work for another. Be patient and willing to adapt your dietary approach based on how your body responds.

Monitor and Adjust: Keep track of your progress and adjust your goals as necessary. Regularly assess whether you're moving in the right direction and make changes based on your experiences.

Celebrate Small Wins: Acknowledge and celebrate your achievements along the way, no matter how small. These mini-celebrations can help maintain motivation.

Stay Informed: Stay informed about the latest research and best practices related to metabolic health and dietary choices. Knowledge can empower you to make informed decisions.

Ultimately, setting realistic goals for a metabolic reset diet involves a combination of science-based knowledge, personalized guidance, and a commitment to gradual, sustainable changes. The emphasis should be on improving your overall health and well-being rather than achieving a quick fix.

CHAPTER FOUR

NUTRITIONAL FOUNDATIONS

Understanding Macronutrients

Understanding macronutrients is crucial when considering metabolic health and its relationship to a "metabolic reset diet." Macronutrients are the essential nutrients that provide energy to the body and are required in relatively large quantities. They include carbohydrates, proteins, and fats. Here's how an understanding of macronutrients relates to metabolism and a metabolic reset diet:

Carbohydrates:

- **Energy Source:** Carbohydrates are the body's primary source of energy. They are broken down into glucose, which fuels various metabolic processes.
- **Role in Metabolism:** Carbohydrates, when consumed in excess, can lead to high blood sugar levels and trigger the release of insulin, a hormone that regulates glucose metabolism.
- **Metabolic Reset:** In the context of a metabolic reset diet, you may focus on consuming complex carbohydrates (e.g., whole grains, vegetables) to provide a steady source of energy, stabilize blood sugar, and improve insulin sensitivity.

Proteins:

Building Blocks: Proteins are essential for building and repairing tissues, including muscle, skin, and enzymes. They also play a role in metabolic processes.

- **Role in Metabolism:** Proteins require energy for digestion and can contribute to the thermic effect of food, which is the energy expended during digestion. This can impact metabolism.
- **Metabolic Reset:** Adequate protein intake is essential to maintain muscle mass, which can support a healthy metabolism. A metabolic reset diet may involve ensuring sufficient protein intake while moderating carbohydrates.

Fats:

Energy Storage: Fats are a concentrated energy source and play a role in the storage of energy for future use.

Role in Metabolism: Dietary fats are essential for the absorption of fat-soluble vitamins (A, D, E, K) and contribute to hormone production.

Metabolic Reset: A balanced intake of healthy fats, such as monounsaturated and polyunsaturated fats, can support overall metabolic health. A metabolic reset diet might involve reducing saturated and trans fats while emphasizing healthy fat sources like avocados, nuts, and fatty fish.

Understanding how these macronutrients are metabolized and their role in metabolic health can help individuals make informed dietary choices. In the context of a metabolic reset diet, the emphasis is often on optimizing macronutrient intake to:

1. Stabilize blood sugar levels by controlling carbohydrate intake and choosing complex carbohydrates.
2. Support muscle mass and metabolic rate through adequate protein consumption.
3. Provide essential fatty acids and support hormone balance through healthy fat choices.

It's important to note that the specific macronutrient ratios that work best for a metabolic reset can vary from person to person, and individual needs should be considered. Consulting with a healthcare professional or registered dietitian is essential for tailoring a metabolic reset diet to your unique requirements and ensuring that it aligns with your metabolic health goals. Additionally, a sustainable and balanced approach to nutrition is generally more effective and conducive to long-term success.

Micronutrients for Metabolism

Micronutrients are essential vitamins and minerals that are required by the body in smaller quantities compared to macronutrients (carbohydrates, proteins, and fats). These micronutrients play a vital role in various metabolic processes that help maintain overall health and well-being. Here are some important micronutrients for metabolism:

1. **Vitamin B Complex:** This group of water-soluble vitamins includes B1 (thiamine), B2 (riboflavin), B3 (niacin), B5 (pantothenic acid), B6 (pyridoxine), B7 (biotin), B9 (folic acid), and B12 (cobalamin). These vitamins are coenzymes that play essential roles in energy metabolism, including the breakdown of carbohydrates, fats, and proteins for energy production.

2. **Vitamin C (Ascorbic Acid):** Vitamin C is necessary for the synthesis of carnitine, a compound that helps transport fatty acids into the mitochondria, where they are metabolized for energy. It also supports the production of certain neurotransmitters and collagen formation.

3. **Vitamin D:** Vitamin D plays a role in calcium metabolism, which is crucial for bone health. It also influences insulin sensitivity and may have an impact on metabolic processes.

4. **Calcium:** Calcium is essential for muscle contraction, including the heart muscle, and plays a role in various

enzymatic reactions, including those involved in energy metabolism.

5. **Magnesium:** Magnesium is a cofactor for more than 300 enzymatic reactions in the body, including those involved in energy production, glucose metabolism, and muscle function.

6. **Iron:** Iron is necessary for the formation of hemoglobin in red blood cells, which carries oxygen to body tissues. Without sufficient iron, energy production can be compromised, leading to fatigue.

7. **Zinc:** Zinc is involved in numerous enzymatic reactions, including those related to carbohydrate and protein metabolism. It also plays a role in insulin function and immune health.

8. **Selenium:** Selenium is a component of selenoproteins, which have antioxidant properties and may help protect cells from oxidative damage related to metabolism.

9. **Copper:** Copper is required for the formation of enzymes involved in energy metabolism, particularly in the mitochondria, where the majority of cellular energy production occurs.

10. **Chromium:** Chromium plays a role in glucose metabolism by enhancing the action of insulin, which helps regulate blood sugar levels.

11. **Manganese:** Manganese is a cofactor for enzymes involved in the metabolism of amino acids, cholesterol, and carbohydrates.

12. **Iodine:** Iodine is essential to produce thyroid hormones, which regulate metabolism. An iodine deficiency can lead to an underactive thyroid and a slower metabolic rate.

These micronutrients can be obtained from a well-balanced diet that includes a variety of foods, such as fruits, vegetables, whole grains, lean proteins, nuts, and seeds. In some cases, dietary supplements may be recommended if an individual has a deficiency or difficulty absorbing specific micronutrients.

Balancing your diet to include a variety of nutrient-rich foods is essential for maintaining overall health and supporting efficient metabolic processes. If you suspect you have a deficiency or are considering dietary supplements, it's advisable to consult with a healthcare professional or registered dietitian for personalized guidance and recommendations.

Hydration and Metabolism

Hydration is closely linked to metabolism and plays a crucial role in various metabolic processes. Here's how hydration affects metabolism:

1. **Cellular Function:** Adequate hydration is essential for optimal cellular function. Water is a primary component of cells, and it plays a role in various biochemical reactions. Without sufficient water, cells may not function properly, which can impact metabolic processes.

2. **Thermoregulation:** The body relies on sweat (primarily composed of water) to cool down and maintain a stable body temperature. When you're dehydrated, your body may struggle to dissipate heat, potentially leading to overheating and an increase in metabolic rate.

3. **Digestion and Nutrient Transport:** Water is necessary for the digestion and absorption of nutrients from the food you eat. It helps break down food in the stomach and small intestine and facilitates the transport of nutrients into the bloodstream.

4. **Blood Circulation:** Proper blood circulation is essential for metabolic processes. Dehydration can lead to reduced blood volume and viscosity, making it more challenging for the circulatory system to deliver oxygen and nutrients to cells and remove waste products.

5. **Energy Production:** The breakdown of macronutrients (carbohydrates, proteins, and fats) for energy production relies on water as a co-factor in enzymatic reactions. Inadequate hydration can hinder the efficiency of these reactions.

6. **Kidney Function:** Hydration is critical for kidney function. The kidneys filter waste products from the blood and maintain electrolyte balance. Dehydration can strain the kidneys and potentially impair their ability to eliminate metabolic waste.

7. **Detoxification:** The body uses water to eliminate waste and toxins through various means, including urine and sweat. Proper hydration supports the body's natural detoxification processes.

8. **Hormone Regulation:** Hormones play a significant role in metabolism. Some hormones, such as vasopressin, are involved in fluid balance and are released in response to hydration status.

9. **Appetite Regulation:** Dehydration can sometimes be mistaken for hunger, leading to overeating. Staying adequately hydrated can help regulate appetite and prevent unnecessary caloric intake.

10. **Weight Management:** Some research suggests that drinking water before meals can enhance weight loss efforts

by promoting a feeling of fullness and reducing the consumption of calories.

It's important to maintain proper hydration for overall health and well-being. Dehydration can lead to a variety of health issues, including reduced physical and mental performance, impaired metabolic function, and an increased risk of kidney stones and urinary tract infections.

The daily water requirements vary from person to person, but a general guideline is to aim for about 8 cups (64 ounces) of water per day. However, individual needs depend on factors like age, activity level, climate, and overall health. Listening to your body and drinking when you're thirsty is an effective way to ensure you stay properly hydrated.

The Role of Fiber

Dietary fiber plays a crucial role in metabolism, particularly in how the body processes and utilizes nutrients. Its effects on metabolism are multifaceted and can have a positive impact on various aspects of health and well-being:

Digestion and Nutrient Absorption: Fiber adds bulk to the diet, aiding in digestion by promoting regular bowel movements and preventing constipation. This can help ensure that the nutrients in the food you consume are efficiently absorbed and utilized.

Blood Sugar Regulation: Soluble fiber, found in foods like oats, beans, and some fruits, can slow the absorption of sugar from the digestive tract into the bloodstream. This helps regulate blood sugar levels and can be particularly beneficial for individuals with diabetes or those at risk of developing it.

Weight Management: Foods high in fiber tend to be more filling and can help control appetite, leading to reduced calorie intake. Fiber-rich foods also require more chewing and take longer to eat, which may promote a feeling of fullness and reduce overall calorie consumption.

Cholesterol Control: Soluble fiber can help lower LDL ("bad") cholesterol levels by binding to cholesterol molecules and removing them from the body. This can reduce the risk of heart disease and support cardiovascular health.

Gut Health: Fiber is prebiotic, which means it serves as a food source for beneficial gut bacteria. A healthy gut microbiome is associated with improved metabolism and overall well-being.

Energy Balance: Fiber helps to slow down the digestion and absorption of carbohydrates, resulting in more stable blood sugar levels and sustained energy. This can be especially important for athletes and those who require long-lasting energy.

Thermogenesis: Dietary fiber, especially from certain foods like whole grains and vegetables, may increase thermogenesis, which is the heat production in the body. This can lead to a slight increase in calorie expenditure during digestion and metabolism.

Healthy Body Weight: A diet rich in fiber can contribute to maintaining a healthy body weight by reducing overall calorie intake, promoting feelings of fullness, and supporting long-term weight management.

It's important to note that there are two main types of dietary fiber: soluble and insoluble fiber. Both types have unique benefits. Soluble fiber dissolves in water and forms a gel-like substance, while insoluble fiber does not dissolve and adds bulk to the diet. A balanced diet should include both types of fiber from a variety of sources, including fruits, vegetables, whole grains, legumes, and nuts.

Incorporating a variety of fiber-rich foods into your diet can help support healthy metabolic processes, improve overall health, and reduce the risk of various chronic diseases. However, it's essential to increase fiber intake gradually and drink plenty of water to prevent digestive discomfort.

CHAPTER FIVE

THE METABOLIC RESET DIET PLAN

Phase 1: Preparing For Reset

In a metabolic reset diet, the preparation phase is crucial as it sets the foundation for a successful reset. During this phase, you'll focus on several key steps to ensure you're ready to make the necessary dietary and lifestyle changes for optimizing your metabolism. Here's an overview of what Phase 1, "Preparing for Reset," might involve:

1. **Goal Setting:** Clearly define your goals and objectives for the metabolic reset. What do you hope to achieve? These goals could be related to weight management, energy levels, blood sugar control, hormonal balance, or other metabolic aspects. Setting specific and achievable goals is essential.

2. **Assessing Current Habits:** Take an honest look at your current dietary and lifestyle habits. What are your typical eating patterns, exercise routines, and stress levels? Identifying areas that need improvement is crucial for making effective changes.

3. **Consultation:** If possible, consult with a healthcare professional or registered dietitian to discuss your goals, assess your current health status, and obtain personalized guidance. They can help you determine the most suitable approach for your metabolic reset.

4. **Meal Planning:** Begin planning meals that align with your metabolic reset goals. Focus on whole, nutrient-dense foods such as vegetables, fruits, lean proteins, whole grains, and healthy fats. Consider portion sizes, meal timing, and nutrient balance.
5. **Pantry Cleanout:** Go through your kitchen and remove or donate processed, unhealthy foods that do not support your reset goals. Stock your pantry and fridge with wholesome, unprocessed options.
6. **Hydration:** Prioritize proper hydration by drinking an adequate amount of water throughout the day. Staying hydrated is essential for metabolic health.
7. **Exercise Plan:** Develop an exercise plan that suits your fitness level and aligns with your metabolic reset goals. Consider a combination of cardiovascular exercises, strength training, and flexibility routines.
8. **Stress Management:** Identify strategies for managing stress, as chronic stress can negatively impact metabolism. This could include techniques like mindfulness, meditation, deep breathing, or yoga.
9. **Sleep Hygiene:** Ensure you are getting sufficient, high-quality sleep. Aim for 7-9 hours of restorative sleep each night to support metabolic health.

10. **Tracking Progress:** Consider methods for tracking your progress during the reset, such as keeping a food journal, using a fitness tracker, or regularly measuring relevant health markers like weight, body composition, and blood sugar levels.

11. **Meal Prep:** Start meal prepping to make it easier to stick to your dietary goals. Having healthy, pre-made meals and snacks on hand can prevent impulsive, less healthy choices.

12. **Support System:** Inform friends and family about your metabolic reset goals and seek their support. Having a support system can make it easier to stay on track.

13. **Educate Yourself:** Take the time to educate yourself about the specific dietary and lifestyle changes you plan to make during the reset. Understanding the reasons behind these changes can enhance motivation and compliance.

14. **Mental Preparedness:** Mental readiness is crucial for a metabolic reset. Be prepared for challenges and setbacks, and develop a positive, resilient mindset to stay motivated.

Phase 1, "Preparing for Reset," sets the stage for a successful metabolic reset diet. It allows you to define your goals, assess your current habits, and make the necessary adjustments to your environment, routines, and support system to ensure a smooth transition into the next phases of the reset.

Eliminating Harmful Foods

Eliminating harmful foods is a crucial step in preparing for a metabolic reset or any health-focused dietary change. The types of harmful foods to be eliminated can vary based on individual health goals and specific dietary plans, but generally, it involves avoiding or significantly reducing the intake of foods that can negatively impact health and metabolism. Here's how to go about eliminating harmful foods:

1. **Identify Harmful Foods:** Start by identifying the foods that are considered harmful for your specific health goals. This may include foods high in added sugars, trans fats, highly processed items, or foods that trigger allergies or sensitivities. Consulting with a healthcare professional or registered dietitian can help pinpoint which foods to eliminate.

2. **Read Food Labels:** Learn to read food labels and ingredient lists. Look for hidden sources of sugar, unhealthy fats, and additives in packaged foods. Avoid products with long lists of artificial ingredients and excessive preservatives.

3. **Reduce Sugary Foods and Drinks:** Added sugars can lead to blood sugar spikes and crashes, weight gain, and other metabolic issues. Eliminate or significantly reduce sugary foods and drinks, including soda, candy, sugary cereals, and heavily sweetened baked goods.

4. **Cut Back on Processed Foods:** Processed foods are often high in sodium, unhealthy fats, and additives. Minimize or eliminate heavily processed items like fast food, packaged snacks, and frozen dinners.

5. **Avoid Trans Fats:** Trans fats, often found in partially hydrogenated oils, can negatively impact cholesterol levels and increase the risk of heart disease. Eliminate foods containing trans fats, such as many fried and baked goods.

6. **Identify Allergens or Sensitivities:** If you have known food allergies or sensitivities, eliminate these foods from your diet. Common allergens include gluten, dairy, peanuts, and shellfish. Avoiding these can help prevent adverse reactions and improve overall health.

7. **Limit Excessive Salt:** High sodium intake can lead to high blood pressure and other health issues. Avoid foods that are excessively high in salt and consider using herbs and spices to flavor your meals instead.

8. **Minimize Refined Grains:** Refined grains like white bread, white rice, and pastries can lead to rapid spikes in blood sugar. Replace them with whole grains like whole wheat bread, brown rice, and quinoa.

9. **Reduce Red and Processed Meats:** High consumption of red and processed meats has been associated with an increased risk of chronic diseases. Limit your intake

and choose lean cuts or alternative protein sources like fish, poultry, beans, and legumes.

10. **Stay Hydrated with Water:** Replace sugary beverages with water as your primary source of hydration. Avoid excessive consumption of sugary drinks, including energy drinks and many fruit juices.

11. **Plan Healthy Substitutes:** Identify healthier alternatives for the harmful foods you're eliminating. This can make the transition easier and more sustainable. For example, swap out sugary desserts for fruit or yogurt.

12. **Prepare Meals at Home:** Cooking your meals at home gives you better control over the ingredients and cooking methods, reducing your exposure to harmful food components.

13. **Educate Yourself:** Learn about the health risks associated with the foods you're eliminating. Understanding the reasons behind these dietary changes can provide motivation and reinforce the importance of your choices.

Remember that eliminating harmful foods doesn't mean you have to completely avoid all indulgences forever. The focus is on making sustainable, long-term changes to improve your health and metabolism. It's important to approach this process with a balanced and realistic mindset and consider seeking guidance from a healthcare professional or registered dietitian for personalized recommendations.

Meal Prep and Planning

Meal prep and planning are integral components of a successful metabolic reset diet or any health-focused dietary change. By carefully planning your meals and preparing them in advance, you can ensure that you have access to nutritious, balanced, and portion-controlled options, which can support your metabolic health and help you stay on track with your goals. Here's how to approach meal prep and planning for a metabolic reset:

1. **Set Clear Goals:** Define your specific dietary and health goals for the metabolic reset. Your goals may include weight management, blood sugar control, hormonal balance, or any other aspect of metabolic health. Having clear objectives will guide your meal planning.

2. **Create a Weekly Menu:** Plan your meals for the week ahead. Consider including a variety of nutrient-dense foods, such as lean proteins, whole grains, plenty of fruits and vegetables, and healthy fats. A balanced menu provides essential nutrients and helps you avoid nutrient deficiencies.

3. **Balance Macronutrients**: Ensure your meals are balanced in terms of macronutrients (carbohydrates, proteins, and fats). This balance can help regulate blood sugar levels, maintain muscle mass, and promote satiety.

4. **Control Portion Sizes:** Be mindful of portion sizes to avoid overeating. Use measuring cups, a food scale, or visual cues to portion out appropriate servings.

5. **Include Fiber:** Integrate fiber-rich foods like whole grains, legumes, and vegetables into your meals. Fiber promotes digestion, helps control appetite, and supports metabolic health.

6. **Plan Snacks:** Include healthy snacks between meals to maintain energy levels and prevent excessive hunger, which can lead to poor food choices. Opt for options like fruit, Greek yogurt, or nuts.

7. **Diversify Protein Sources:** Include a variety of protein sources in your meals, such as lean meats, poultry, fish, beans, lentils, tofu, and dairy products. Protein is essential for muscle maintenance and can support metabolic rate.

8. **Prepare Ahead of Time:** Dedicate a specific time each week to meal preparation. Cook and portion your meals and snacks for the coming days, making them easily accessible when you need them.

9. **Use the Right Tools:** Invest in quality storage containers to keep your prepared meals fresh. You may also want to use a meal planner or a smartphone app to organize your weekly menu.

10. **Label and Date:** To avoid confusion, label your containers with the date they were prepared and the contents. This will help you identify the freshness of your meals.

11. **Refrigerate or Freeze:** Store your prepared meals in the refrigerator or freezer, depending on when you plan to consume them. Freezing can extend the shelf life of prepared dishes.

12. **Plan for Variety:** Ensure your meals are enjoyable and satisfying by incorporating a range of flavors, textures, and cuisines. Variety can prevent dietary boredom and help you stick to your plan.

13. **Review and Adjust:** Periodically review your meal plan and adjust it based on your progress and feedback from your body. Be open to making necessary changes to better meet your metabolic reset goals.

14. **Stay Hydrated:** Don't forget to include adequate water intake in your meal plan. Proper hydration is essential for metabolism and overall health.

Meal prep and planning help you avoid impulsive and unhealthy food choices, making it easier to stick to your metabolic reset diet. It can save you time and money while promoting better health outcomes. Remember that flexibility is key, and it's okay to adapt your plan as needed to accommodate changing circumstances and preferences.

Phase 2: Resetting Your Metabolism

In Phase 2 of resetting your metabolism, you'll begin to implement the dietary and lifestyle changes you prepared for in Phase 1. This phase is the heart of your metabolic reset journey, where you'll take active steps to optimize your metabolism. Here's how Phase 2, "Resetting Your Metabolism," typically unfolds:

1. **Follow Your Prepared Meal Plan:** Stick to the meal plan you created in Phase 1. Ensure your meals are well-balanced and aligned with your metabolic reset goals.

2. **Portion Control:** Pay attention to portion sizes. Be mindful of what you're eating and aim to control calorie intake based on your metabolic goals, whether it's weight loss, maintenance, or other objectives.

3. **Prioritize Nutrient-Dense Foods:** Continue to prioritize nutrient-dense foods such as fruits, vegetables, lean proteins, whole grains, and healthy fats. These foods provide essential vitamins, minerals, and fiber to support metabolic health.

4. **Hydration:** Maintain proper hydration by drinking an adequate amount of water throughout the day. Staying hydrated is essential for metabolic processes.

5. **Regular Meal Timing:** Stick to regular mealtimes to help regulate blood sugar levels and prevent excessive hunger. Eating at consistent intervals can support metabolic stability.

6. **Balanced Macronutrients:** Ensure that your meals contain a balance of carbohydrates, proteins, and healthy fats to support energy production and overall metabolic health.

7. **Reduce Sugar Intake:** Continue to minimize added sugars in your diet. Be vigilant about reading food labels and avoid sugary snacks and drinks.

8. **Manage Stress:** Implement stress management techniques such as mindfulness, meditation, or relaxation exercises. Reducing stress is crucial for metabolic health.

9. **Regular Exercise:** Adhere to your exercise plan established in Phase 1. Regular physical activity can help boost metabolism, improve insulin sensitivity, and support weight management.

10. **Quality Sleep:** Continue to prioritize quality sleep. Aim for 7-9 hours of restorative sleep each night to support metabolic health.

11. **Monitor Progress:** Track your progress by measuring relevant health markers, such as weight, body composition,

blood sugar levels, and energy levels. Monitoring your progress can help you stay on course and adjust as needed.

12. **Seek Support:** Lean on your support system, whether it's friends, family, or a support group. Share your experiences, seek encouragement, and hold yourself accountable.

13. **Educate Yourself:** Continue to educate yourself about the reasons behind the dietary and lifestyle changes you're making. Knowledge can strengthen your commitment and motivation.

14. **Stay Mindful:** Be mindful of your food choices, emotional eating triggers, and any deviations from your meal plan. Developing a heightened awareness of your eating habits can help you make healthier choices.

15. **Adapt as Needed:** Be prepared to adapt your plan as your metabolic reset progresses. Listen to your body and respond to its feedback to make the necessary adjustments.

This phase of your metabolic reset may last several weeks to several months, depending on your individual goals and progress. The key is consistency, patience, and a long-term commitment to maintaining a healthier lifestyle. Remember that metabolic reset diets are not quick fixes but rather a holistic approach to optimizing your metabolism and improving overall health.

Meal Timing Strategies

Meal timing is an important aspect of a metabolic reset diet, and the timing of your meals and snacks can impact your energy levels, blood sugar control, and overall metabolic health. Here are some meal timing strategies to consider during your metabolic reset:

1. **Regular Meal Schedule:** Stick to a regular meal schedule by eating meals at approximately the same times each day. This consistency helps regulate your circadian rhythm and can improve metabolic function.

2. **Balanced Breakfast:** Start your day with a balanced breakfast that includes protein, complex carbohydrates, and healthy fats. Breakfast provides energy and can help stabilize blood sugar levels, reducing the risk of overeating later in the day.

3. **Frequent, Smaller Meals:** Some people find it beneficial to eat smaller, more frequent meals throughout the day, rather than three large meals. This approach can help maintain steady energy levels and prevent overeating.

4. **Intuitive Eating:** Listen to your body's hunger and fullness cues. Eat when you're hungry and stop when you're satisfied. This intuitive approach to eating can help prevent excessive calorie intake.

5. **Protein Timing:** Include a source of protein in each of your meals. Protein can promote satiety and help maintain muscle mass, which is important for metabolism.

6. **Post-Workout Nutrition:** If you exercise, consider consuming a combination of protein and carbohydrates after your workout to support muscle recovery and replenish glycogen stores.

7. **Mid-Morning and Afternoon Snacks:** Include healthy snacks between meals to prevent energy dips and excessive hunger. Opt for nutrient-dense options like fruit, Greek yogurt, or nuts.

8. **Early Dinner:** Aim to have dinner at least a few hours before bedtime. Eating too close to bedtime can disrupt sleep and may negatively affect metabolism.

9. **Avoid Late-Night Snacking:** Avoid snacking late at night, as this can interfere with sleep quality and lead to excessive calorie intake.

10. **Time-Restricted Eating:** Consider implementing a time-restricted eating pattern, where you limit your food intake to a specific window of hours each day. This can support circadian rhythms and improve metabolic health.

11. **Avoid Skipping Meals:** Skipping meals can lead to irregular blood sugar levels and overeating later in the day. Try to have regular, balanced meals.

12. **Monitor Your Body's Response:** Pay attention to how your body responds to different meal timing strategies. Some people may function better with a traditional three-meals-a-day approach, while others may prefer intermittent fasting or other patterns.

13. **Stay Hydrated:** Don't forget to hydrate between meals. Proper hydration is essential for metabolic processes and can sometimes be confused with hunger.

14. **Consult a Dietitian:** If you have specific dietary needs or medical conditions, consider consulting a registered dietitian or healthcare professional. They can help you create a personalized meal timing strategy tailored to your unique requirements.

Meal timing can be highly individual, and what works best for one person may not work for another. Experiment with different strategies, pay attention to how your body responds, and be flexible in adjusting your meal timing to best support your metabolic reset goals.

Intermittent Fasting

Intermittent fasting is an eating pattern that involves cycling between periods of fasting and eating. It has gained popularity for its potential health benefits, including improved metabolic health. There are several methods of intermittent fasting, and individuals can choose the one that best aligns with their preferences and goals. Here are some common intermittent fasting methods:

16/8 Method: This method involves fasting for 16 hours each day and restricting your eating to an 8-hour window. For example, you might eat between 12:00 PM and 8:00 PM and fast from 8:00 PM to 12:00 PM the following day.

5:2 Diet: In this approach, you consume your regular diet for five days of the week and restrict your calorie intake to about 500-600 calories on the remaining two non-consecutive days.

Eat-Stop-Eat: With this method, you fast for a full 24 hours once or twice a week. For example, you might eat dinner one day and not eat again until dinner the following day.

Alternate-Day Fasting: On alternate days, you either fast completely or significantly reduce your calorie intake. On non-fasting days, you eat normally.

The Warrior Diet: This method involves fasting for 20 hours and having a 4-hour eating window in the evening. During the fasting period, you can consume small amounts of raw fruits and vegetables.

OMAD (One Meal a Day): With OMAD, you fast for approximately 23 hours and consume all your daily calories within a one-hour eating window.

Intermittent fasting may offer several potential benefits related to metabolism and overall health:

- Weight Management: Intermittent fasting can help control calorie intake, leading to weight loss or weight maintenance. It may also promote the loss of body fat while preserving lean muscle mass.

- Blood Sugar Control: Fasting periods can improve insulin sensitivity, regulate blood sugar levels, and reduce the risk of type 2 diabetes.

- Improved Lipid Profile: Some studies suggest that intermittent fasting can reduce triglycerides and LDL ("bad") cholesterol levels, improving heart health.

- Cellular Health: Fasting triggers cellular repair processes and autophagy, which remove damaged components, supporting overall cell health.

- Longevity: Animal studies have shown that intermittent fasting may extend lifespan and improve aging-related health markers.

- Brain Health: Some research suggests that intermittent fasting may support brain health by enhancing the production of brain-derived neurotrophic factor (BDNF) and reducing oxidative stress.

It's important to note that intermittent fasting is not suitable for everyone. It may not be appropriate for individuals with certain medical conditions, pregnant or breastfeeding women, or those with a history of eating disorders. If you're considering intermittent fasting, it's advisable to consult with a healthcare professional or registered dietitian to ensure it aligns with your health goals and that you're following a safe and sustainable approach. Additionally, it's essential to stay hydrated during fasting periods and focus on nutritious, balanced meals during eating windows to support your overall health and metabolism.

Phase 3: Maintaining A Healthy Metabolism

Phase 3, "Maintaining a Healthy Metabolism," is the long-term continuation of your metabolic reset journey. After the initial phases of preparation and active resetting, this phase focuses on sustaining the positive changes you've made and ensuring your metabolism remains in a healthy state. Here's how to approach this phase:

1. **Lifestyle Integration:** View the metabolic reset changes you've made as part of your new, sustainable lifestyle. These are not temporary measures but long-term habits that support your health.

2. **Consistency:** Consistency is key. Continue to follow the dietary and lifestyle habits that you've established during the reset. Consistency helps maintain a healthy metabolism.

3. **Regular Monitoring:** Periodically monitor your health markers, such as weight, body composition, blood sugar levels, and other relevant metrics. This helps you track your progress and adjust if needed.

4. **Adapt to Changes:** Be flexible and adaptable. Life circumstances and goals may change, so be open to modifying your dietary and exercise plans to accommodate these changes.

5. **Support System:** Continue to rely on your support system for encouragement and motivation. Share your

experiences and successes with friends and family who are supporting your journey.

6. **Education:** Stay informed about the latest research and guidelines related to metabolic health. Education ensures that you can adjust your strategies as new information becomes available.

7. **Mindful Eating:** Maintain mindful eating habits. Be attentive to hunger and fullness cues and make informed choices about the foods you consume.

8. **Hydration:** Continue to prioritize proper hydration. Drinking enough water is essential for metabolic health.

9. **Physical Activity:** Keep up with regular physical activity. Maintain your exercise routine to support muscle mass, metabolic rate, and overall well-being.

10. **Stress Management:** Continue to practice stress management techniques to keep stress levels in check. Chronic stress can negatively impact metabolism.

11. **Quality Sleep:** Prioritize quality sleep for at least 7-9 hours per night. Sleep plays a significant role in metabolic health.

12. **Nutrient-Dense Foods:** Emphasize nutrient-dense foods in your diet. Continue to consume a variety of fruits, vegetables, lean proteins, whole grains, and healthy fats.
13. **Occasional Indulgences:** It's realistic to enjoy occasional indulgences but maintain moderation in your approach. Special treats can be part of a balanced lifestyle.

14. **Regular Health Checkups:** Schedule regular checkups with a healthcare professional to assess your overall health, address any concerns, and track your metabolic health.

15. **Plan for Challenges:** Anticipate and plan for potential challenges and setbacks. Develop strategies to overcome obstacles and stay on track.

16. **Long-Term Mindset:** Think about your metabolic reset as a lifelong journey. The goal is to maintain a healthy metabolism and overall well-being over the years.

It's important to understand that metabolic health is not a one-time achievement but an ongoing process. The habits and choices you've cultivated during the reset phase are meant to be sustainable and adaptable as you navigate life's changes. With a long-term commitment to maintaining a healthy metabolism, you can enjoy improved health, sustained energy, and an enhanced quality of life.

Long-Term Nutrition Strategies

Long-term nutrition strategies are crucial for maintaining a healthy metabolism and overall well-being over the years. These strategies involve sustainable, balanced eating habits that promote optimal health, support your metabolic goals, and can be maintained for a lifetime. Here are some long-term nutrition strategies to consider:

1. **Whole, Unprocessed Foods:** Base your diet on whole, unprocessed foods. These include fruits, vegetables, whole grains, lean proteins, and healthy fats. These foods are rich in nutrients and support metabolic health.

2. **Portion Control:** Pay attention to portion sizes to avoid overeating. Be mindful of how much you eat and avoid excessive calorie consumption.

3. **Balanced Macronutrients:** Consume a balance of carbohydrates, proteins, and healthy fats at each meal. This balance supports energy production and metabolic stability.

4. **Fiber-Rich Foods:** Continue to include fiber-rich foods in your diet. Fiber aids digestion, promotes satiety, and helps control blood sugar levels.

5. **Protein Variety:** Include a variety of protein sources in your diet, such as lean meats, poultry, fish, beans, lentils, tofu, and dairy products. Protein is essential for muscle maintenance and metabolism.

6. **Limit Sugars and Processed Foods:** Minimize the intake of added sugars and highly processed foods. These can lead to blood sugar spikes, weight gain, and other metabolic issues.

7. **Healthy Fats:** Incorporate sources of healthy fats like avocados, nuts, seeds, and olive oil into your diet. These fats support heart health and overall well-being.

8. **Regular Meal Timing:** Maintain regular meal timing to help regulate blood sugar levels and prevent excessive hunger.

9. **Hydration:** Continue to prioritize proper hydration by drinking an adequate amount of water throughout the day.

10. **Mindful Eating:** Be mindful of your food choices and eating habits. Pay attention to hunger and fullness cues and make informed decisions about what you consume.

11. **Variety and Moderation**: Embrace variety in your diet and enjoy a wide range of foods. Moderation is key when it comes to occasional indulgences.

12. **Meal Planning:** Continue meal planning and preparation to ensure you have access to healthy, balanced options that align with your metabolic goals.

13. **Nutrition Education:** Stay informed about the latest nutritional research and guidelines. Knowledge empowers you to make informed choices about your diet.

14. **Long-Term Goals:** Think about your nutrition as a long-term commitment to health and well-being. The goal is to maintain a healthy metabolism and overall quality of life.

15. **Regular Health Checkups:** Schedule regular checkups with a healthcare professional to assess your overall health, address any concerns, and track your metabolic health.

16. **Adapt to Life Changes:** Life circumstances and goals may change, so be open to adjusting your nutrition strategies as needed to accommodate these changes.

17. **Family and Social Support:** Involve your family and social circles in your nutrition plan. Encourage healthy eating together and seek support from loved ones.

18. **Seek Professional Guidance:** If you have specific dietary needs or medical conditions, consider consulting with a registered dietitian or healthcare professional for personalized guidance.

Remember that the key to long-term nutrition strategies is sustainability and flexibility. Your eating habits should be adaptable to accommodate changes in your life while supporting your metabolic health and overall well-being. A balanced, whole-foods-based approach to nutrition is not only effective for metabolism but can also enhance your overall quality of life.

Transitioning Out of Reset Mode

Transitioning out of the reset phase is an important step in a metabolic reset diet. It involves moving from the structured, active phase of resetting your metabolism to a more flexible, long-term approach to maintaining your health. Here's how to transition effectively:

Gradual Adjustments: Avoid abrupt changes to your dietary and lifestyle habits. Gradually reintroduce foods or behaviors that were restricted during the reset phase but do so mindfully.

Monitoring: Continue to monitor your progress and health markers, even as you transition out of the reset phase. This helps you ensure that your metabolic health remains on track.

Balance: Maintain a balanced approach to your diet. Continue to prioritize nutrient-dense, whole foods, but allow room for occasional indulgences without guilt.

Consistency: Keep up with the healthy habits you've established during the reset phase. Consistency is key to long-term success.

Flexibility: Adapt to changes in your life, schedule, and goals. Be flexible in adjusting your dietary and exercise plans as needed.

Education: Stay informed about the latest research and guidelines related to metabolic health. Knowledge empowers you to make informed choices about your diet and lifestyle.

Regular Health Checkups: Continue scheduling regular checkups with a healthcare professional to assess your overall health, address any concerns, and track your metabolic health.

Support System: Maintain your support system for encouragement and motivation. Share your experiences and successes with friends and family who are supporting your journey.

Mindful Eating: Continue practicing mindful eating habits. Be attentive to hunger and fullness cues and make informed choices about the foods you consume.

Stress Management: Keep practicing stress management techniques to keep stress levels in check. Chronic stress can negatively impact metabolism.

Quality Sleep: Prioritize quality sleep for at least 7-9 hours per night. Sleep plays a significant role in metabolic health.

Physical Activity: Maintain your regular exercise routine to support muscle mass, metabolic rate, and overall well-being.

Variety: Embrace variety in your diet and enjoy a wide range of foods. Moderation is key when it comes to occasional indulgences.

Educate Others: Share your experience and knowledge with others who may benefit from a metabolic reset. Encourage healthy eating and lifestyle habits within your social circles.

Adaptive Goals: Adjust your goals as needed based on your progress and life circumstances. Your metabolic health journey is a long-term commitment.

The transition phase is an opportunity to fine-tune your approach and develop a sustainable, lifelong commitment to a healthy lifestyle. Continue to make choices that support your metabolic health while enjoying a well-rounded and balanced approach to eating and living.

Week-By-Week Meal Plans For Each Phase

Creating week-by-week meal plans for each phase of a metabolic reset diet can help you stay organized and on track with your goals. Here are sample meal plans for each phase: Preparation (Phase 1), Reset (Phase 2), and Maintenance (Phase 3).

PHASE 1: PREPARATION

During the preparation phase, you're setting the stage for your metabolic reset. Focus on cleaning up your diet and creating a foundation for the upcoming phases.

Week 1:

Day 1:

Breakfast: Oatmeal with berries and a sprinkle of nuts.

Lunch: Grilled chicken salad with mixed greens and a vinaigrette dressing.

Dinner: Baked salmon with quinoa and steamed broccoli.

Day 2:

Breakfast: Greek yogurt with honey and sliced bananas.

Lunch: Turkey and avocado wrap with whole-grain tortilla.

Dinner: Stir-fried tofu with mixed vegetables and brown rice.

Day 3:

Breakfast: Scrambled eggs with spinach and tomatoes.

Lunch: Lentil soup and a side salad.

Dinner: Baked cod with sweet potato and asparagus.

Day 4:

Breakfast: Whole-grain cereal with low-fat milk and sliced strawberries.

Lunch: Grilled vegetable and hummus wrap.

Dinner: Baked chicken breast with quinoa and roasted asparagus.

Day 5:

Breakfast: Smoothie with spinach, banana, almond milk, and a scoop of protein powder.

Lunch: Lentil and vegetable soup with a side of mixed greens.

Dinner: Grilled tilapia with brown rice and steamed green beans.

Day 6:

Breakfast: Oatmeal with sliced peaches and a sprinkle of almonds.

Lunch: Turkey and avocado salad with mixed greens and balsamic dressing.

Dinner: Stir-fried tofu with mixed vegetables and quinoa.

Day 7:

Breakfast: Scrambled eggs with diced bell peppers and whole-grain toast.

Lunch: Chickpea and cucumber salad with a lemon-tahini dressing.

Dinner: Baked pork tenderloin with sweet potato and broccoli.

These meal plans provide a variety of nutrient-dense foods, setting the foundation for a successful metabolic reset in Phase 2. Remember to adjust the portion sizes and specific foods based on your dietary preferences and any individual health needs.

PHASE 2: RESET

In Phase 2, you're actively resetting your metabolism with specific dietary and lifestyle changes.

Week 2:

Day 1:

Breakfast: A vegetable omelet with a side of mixed berries.

Lunch: Quinoa salad with chickpeas, cucumber, and feta cheese.

Dinner: Grilled chicken breast with roasted Brussels sprouts and brown rice.

Day 2:

Breakfast: Greek yogurt with chia seeds and a drizzle of honey.

Lunch: Spinach and kale salad with grilled shrimp and a citrus vinaigrette.

Dinner: Baked trout with quinoa and steamed asparagus.

Day 3:

Breakfast: Overnight oats with almond butter and sliced apples.

Lunch: Lentil and vegetable stir-fry with tofu.

Dinner: Grilled sirloin steak with roasted sweet potatoes and green beans.

Day 4:

Breakfast: Greek yogurt with sliced peaches and a drizzle of honey.

Lunch: Spinach and arugula salad with grilled chicken and a balsamic vinaigrette.

Dinner: Baked cod with quinoa and roasted asparagus.

Day 5:

Breakfast: Scrambled eggs with spinach and diced tomatoes.

Lunch: Quinoa and black bean salad with avocado.

Dinner: Grilled salmon with brown rice and sautéed green beans.

Day 6:

Breakfast: Smoothie with kale, banana, almond milk, and chia seeds.

Lunch: Lentil and vegetable stir-fry with tofu.

Dinner: Grilled sirloin steak with sweet potato and mixed greens.

Day 7:

Breakfast: Oatmeal with mixed berries and a dollop of Greek yogurt.

Lunch: Mixed greens salad with shrimp and a citrus vinaigrette.

Dinner: Baked trout with quinoa and steamed broccoli.

These meal plans continue to emphasize nutrient-dense foods, portion control, and balanced macronutrients to support your metabolic reset in Phase 2. Adjust the specific foods to suit your preferences and dietary requirements.

PHASE 3: MAINTENANCE

Phase 3 is about maintaining a healthy metabolism and incorporating the changes you made in Phase 2 into your long-term lifestyle.

Week 3:

Day 1:

Breakfast: Whole-grain toast with avocado and poached eggs.

Lunch: Spinach and strawberry salad with grilled chicken and balsamic dressing.

Dinner: Baked cod with quinoa and sautéed spinach.

Day 2:

Breakfast: Smoothie with spinach, banana, Greek yogurt, and almond milk.

Lunch: Lentil and vegetable soup with a side of mixed greens.

Dinner: Grilled salmon with brown rice and roasted broccoli.

Day 3:

Breakfast: Scrambled eggs with diced tomatoes, peppers, and onions.

Lunch: Turkey and hummus wrap with a side of carrot sticks.

Dinner: Stir-fried tofu with quinoa and steamed green beans.

Day 4:

Breakfast: Whole-grain waffles with almond butter and sliced strawberries.

Lunch: Spinach and walnut salad with grilled chicken and a vinaigrette dressing.

Dinner: Baked cod with quinoa and steamed asparagus.

Day 5:

Breakfast: Greek yogurt with honey and mixed berries.

Lunch: Lentil and vegetable stir-fry with tofu.

Dinner: Grilled salmon with brown rice and sautéed green beans.

Day 6:

Breakfast: Scrambled eggs with spinach and sliced tomatoes.

Lunch: Turkey and hummus wrap with a side of carrot sticks.

Dinner: Baked pork tenderloin with sweet potato and mixed greens.

Day 7:

Breakfast: Smoothie with kale, banana, almond milk, and a scoop of protein powder.

Lunch: Chickpea and cucumber salad with a lemon-tahini dressing.

Dinner: Grilled trout with quinoa and roasted broccoli.

These meal plans aim to maintain the healthy eating habits established during the reset phase in Phase 2 while offering flexibility and enjoyment. Feel free to adjust the specific foods and portion sizes according to your preferences and dietary requirements.

These are just sample meal plans to give you an idea of how to structure your meals in each phase. Your actual meal plans should be tailored to your individual goals, preferences, dietary restrictions, and calorie needs. Consider working with a registered dietitian to create personalized meal plans that suit your specific metabolic reset objectives.

BALANCED AND DELICIOUS RECIPES

Here are five balanced and delicious breakfast recipes, along with instructions and nutritional information for each one:

BREAKFAST:

1. Greek Yogurt Parfait

Ingredients:

1 cup Greek yogurt

1/2 cup mixed berries (strawberries, blueberries, raspberries)

2 tablespoons honey

1/4 cup granola (optional)

Instructions:

In a serving bowl or glass, start with a layer of Greek yogurt.

Add a layer of mixed berries.

Drizzle honey over the berries.

Repeat the layers as desired.

Top with granola for added crunch (optional).

Nutritional Information (per serving):

Calories: 350

Protein: 20g

Carbohydrates: 45g

Fiber: 5g

Sugars: 28g

Fat: 11g

Saturated Fat: 3g

2. Spinach and Feta Omelette

Ingredients:

2 large eggs

1 cup fresh spinach, chopped

2 tablespoons feta cheese

Salt and pepper to taste

Cooking spray or olive oil for the pan

Instructions:

Whisk the eggs in a bowl and season with salt and pepper.

Heat a non-stick skillet over medium heat and lightly grease it.

Pour the eggs into the skillet.

Add chopped spinach and crumbled feta to one-half of the omelet.

Fold the other half of the omelet over the filling.

Cook until the eggs are set, about 2-3 minutes on each side.

Nutritional Information (per serving):

Calories: 230

Protein: 16g

Carbohydrates: 3g

Fiber: 1g

Sugars: 1g

Fat: 17g

Saturated Fat: 7g

3. Peanut Butter Banana Smoothie

Ingredients:

1 ripe banana

2 tablespoons natural peanut butter

1 cup unsweetened almond milk

1/2 cup Greek yogurt

1 teaspoon honey (optional)

Ice cubes (as desired)

Instructions:

Place all ingredients in a blender.

Blend until smooth and creamy.

Add more almond milk if a thinner consistency is desired.

Nutritional Information (per serving):

Calories: 340

Protein: 16g

Carbohydrates: 29g

Fiber: 4g

Sugars: 15g

Fat: 20g

Saturated Fat: 3g

4. Veggie and Cheese Breakfast Quesadilla

Ingredients:

2 small whole-grain tortillas

2 large eggs, scrambled

1/2 cup diced bell peppers

1/4 cup shredded cheddar cheese

Salt and pepper to taste

Cooking spray

Instructions:

Heat a non-stick skillet over medium heat and lightly grease it.

Place one tortilla in the skillet.

Sprinkle half of the cheese on the tortilla.

Add scrambled eggs and diced bell peppers.

Sprinkle the remaining cheese on top.

Place the second tortilla on top.

Cook until the quesadilla is golden brown, then flip and cook the other side.

Nutritional Information (per serving):

Calories: 350

Protein: 20g

Carbohydrates: 31g

Fiber: 7g

Sugars: 4g

Fat: 16g / Saturated Fat: 6g

5. Overnight Chia Pudding

Ingredients:

2 tablespoons chia seeds

1 cup unsweetened almond milk

1/2 teaspoon vanilla extract

1 tablespoon maple syrup or honey

Fresh berries for topping

Instructions:

In a jar or bowl, combine chia seeds, almond milk, vanilla extract, and maple syrup or honey.

Stir well, ensuring the chia seeds are fully mixed in.

Cover and refrigerate overnight (or for at least 4 hours).

In the morning, top with fresh berries before serving.

Nutritional Information (per serving):

Calories: 210

Protein: 6g

Carbohydrates: 23g

Fiber: 10g

Sugars: 11g

Fat: 11g

Saturated Fat: 1g

These breakfast recipes offer a variety of flavors and nutrients while keeping your first meal of the day balanced and delicious. Enjoy!

LUNCH RECIPES:

Here are five balanced and delicious lunch recipes, along with instructions and nutritional information for each one:

1. Grilled Chicken and Quinoa Salad

Ingredients:

4 oz grilled chicken breast, sliced

1 cup cooked quinoa

2 cups mixed greens (e.g., spinach, arugula, kale)

1/4 cup cherry tomatoes, halved

1/4 cup cucumber, sliced

2 tablespoons balsamic vinaigrette

Instructions:

In a large bowl, arrange the mixed greens.

Top with sliced grilled chicken, cooked quinoa, cherry tomatoes, and cucumber.

Drizzle balsamic vinaigrette over the salad.

Toss to combine and serve.

Nutritional Information (per serving):

Calories: 400

Protein: 30g

Carbohydrates: 35g

Fiber: 5g / Sugars: 4g

Fat: 16g / Saturated Fat: 2g

2. Chickpea and Avocado Wrap

Ingredients:

1 whole-grain tortilla

1/2 cup canned chickpeas, drained and mashed

1/2 avocado, sliced

1/4 cup mixed greens

2 tablespoons hummus

Salt and pepper to taste

Instructions:

Lay the whole-grain tortilla flat.

Spread mashed chickpeas and hummus evenly.

Layer on sliced avocado and mixed greens.

Season with salt and pepper.

Roll up the tortilla, slice in half, and serve.

Nutritional Information (per serving):

Calories: 380

Protein: 10g

Carbohydrates: 44g

Fiber: 13g

Sugars: 2g

Fat: 19g

Saturated Fat: 3g

3. Salmon and Quinoa Bowl

Ingredients:

4 oz baked or grilled salmon

1 cup cooked quinoa

1 cup steamed broccoli florets

1/4 cup shredded carrots

1 tablespoon soy sauce or tamari

1/2 teaspoon sesame seeds

Instructions:

In a bowl, layer the cooked quinoa.

Add the steamed broccoli and shredded carrots.

Place the salmon on top.

Drizzle with soy sauce and sprinkle sesame seeds.

Serve warm.

Nutritional Information (per serving):

Calories: 380

Protein: 30g

Carbohydrates: 35g

Fiber: 6g

Sugars: 2g

Fat: 14g

Saturated Fat: 2g

4. Lentil and Vegetable Stir-Fry

Ingredients:

1 cup cooked green or brown lentils

1 cup mixed vegetables (e.g., bell peppers, broccoli, snap peas)

2 tablespoons low-sodium stir-fry sauce

1 tablespoon olive oil

2 tablespoons sliced almonds

Instructions:

Heat olive oil in a skillet over medium-high heat.

Add the mixed vegetables and stir-fry for 3-4 minutes.

Add cooked lentils and stir-fry sauce. Cook for an additional 2-3 minutes.

Top with sliced almonds and serve.

Nutritional Information (per serving):

Calories: 350

Protein: 15g

Carbohydrates: 45g

Fiber: 12g

Sugars: 3g

Fat: 12g

Saturated Fat: 1g

5. Caprese Salad with Grilled Chicken

Ingredients:

4 oz grilled chicken breast, sliced

1 cup cherry tomatoes, halved

1 cup fresh mozzarella cheese, cubed

1/4 cup fresh basil leaves

1 tablespoon balsamic glaze

Salt and pepper to taste

Instructions:

In a large bowl, combine cherry tomatoes, mozzarella, and fresh basil leaves.

Top with sliced grilled chicken.

Drizzle with balsamic glaze and season with salt and pepper.

Toss to combine and serve.

Nutritional Information (per serving):

Calories: 430

Protein: 30g

Carbohydrates: 5g

Fiber: 1g

Sugars: 3g

Fat: 30g

Saturated Fat: 15g

These lunch recipes offer a variety of flavors and nutrients while keeping your midday meal balanced and delicious. Enjoy!

DINNER RECIPES:

Here are five balanced and delicious dinner recipes, along with instructions and nutritional information for each one:

1. Baked Salmon with Quinoa and Asparagus

Ingredients:

4 oz baked or grilled salmon

1 cup cooked quinoa

1 cup steamed asparagus

1 tablespoon olive oil

Lemon juice and zest

Salt and pepper to taste

Instructions:

Place the cooked quinoa on a plate.

Top with steamed asparagus and baked salmon.

Drizzle with olive oil and lemon juice.

Season with salt, pepper, and lemon zest.

Serve hot.

Nutritional Information (per serving):

Calories: 380

Protein: 30g

Carbohydrates: 30g

Fiber: 5g / Sugars: 2g

Fat: 16g / Saturated Fat: 3g

2. Vegetable Stir-Fry with Tofu

Ingredients:

1 cup firm tofu, cubed

2 cups mixed vegetables (e.g., bell peppers, broccoli, carrots)

2 tablespoons low-sodium stir-fry sauce

1 tablespoon sesame oil

1 cup cooked brown rice

Instructions:

Heat sesame oil in a wok or skillet over medium-high heat.

Add tofu and stir-fry for 3-4 minutes until lightly browned.

Add mixed vegetables and stir-fry sauce. Cook for an additional 4-5 minutes.

Serve over cooked brown rice.

Nutritional Information (per serving):

Calories: 410

Protein: 18g

Carbohydrates: 40g

Fiber: 6g

Sugars: 3g

Fat: 18g

Saturated Fat: 3g

3. Grilled Chicken with Sweet Potato and Green Beans

Ingredients:

4 oz grilled chicken breast

1 medium sweet potato, roasted

1 cup steamed green beans

1 tablespoon olive oil

Garlic powder, paprika, and salt to taste

Instructions:

Season the chicken with garlic powder, paprika, and salt.

Grill the chicken until cooked through.

Serve with roasted sweet potato and steamed green beans.

Drizzle with olive oil and season with additional salt if desired.

Nutritional Information (per serving):

Calories: 420

Protein: 35g

Carbohydrates: 40g

Fiber: 8g

Sugars: 9g

Fat: 15g

Saturated Fat: 2g

4. Lentil and Vegetable Soup

Ingredients:

1 cup cooked green or brown lentils

2 cups vegetable broth

1 cup mixed vegetables (e.g., carrots, celery, onions)

1 clove garlic, minced

1 teaspoon olive oil

Salt and pepper to taste

Instructions:

Heat olive oil in a soup pot over medium heat.

Add minced garlic and mixed vegetables. Sauté for 5-6 minutes.

Add cooked lentils and vegetable broth.

Simmer for 15-20 minutes until the vegetables are tender.

Season with salt and pepper before serving.

Nutritional Information (per serving):

Calories: 360

Protein: 18g

Carbohydrates: 60g

Fiber: 15g

Sugars: 6g

Fat: 6g

Saturated Fat: 1g

5. Quinoa and Black Bean Stuffed Bell Peppers

Ingredients:

2 bell peppers, halved and deseeded

1 cup cooked quinoa

1 cup canned black beans, rinsed and drained

1 cup salsa

1/2 cup shredded cheddar cheese

1 teaspoon chili powder

Salt and pepper to taste

Instructions:

Preheat the oven to 375°F (190°C).

In a bowl, mix quinoa, black beans, salsa, chili powder, salt, and pepper.

Stuff the bell pepper halves with the quinoa mixture.

Place in a baking dish, cover with foil, and bake for 30 minutes.

Remove the foil, sprinkle with cheddar cheese, and bake for an additional 10 minutes.

Nutritional Information (per serving):

Calories: 420

Protein: 18g

Carbohydrates: 68g

Fiber: 14g

Sugars: 7g

Fat: 9g

Saturated Fat: 4g

These dinner recipes provide a variety of flavors and nutrients while keeping your evening meal balanced and delicious. Enjoy!

SNACKS RECIPES:

Here are five balanced and delicious snack recipes, along with instructions and nutritional information for each one:

1. Greek Yogurt and Berry Parfait

Ingredients:

1 cup Greek yogurt

1/2 cup mixed berries (strawberries, blueberries, raspberries)

2 tablespoons honey

2 tablespoons granola (optional)

Instructions:

In a glass or bowl, start with a layer of Greek yogurt.

Add a layer of mixed berries.

Drizzle honey over the berries.

Repeat the layers as desired.

Top with granola for added crunch (optional).

Nutritional Information (per serving):

Calories: 250

Protein: 15g

Carbohydrates: 35g

Fiber: 4g

Sugars: 26g

Fat: 5g

Saturated Fat: 0.5g

2. Hummus and Veggie Snack Plate

Ingredients:

2 tablespoons hummus

Baby carrots

Cherry tomatoes

Cucumber slices

Bell pepper strips

Instructions:

Arrange the hummus in a small bowl or container.

Surround it with baby carrots, cherry tomatoes, cucumber slices, and bell pepper strips.

Dip the veggies in hummus for a tasty and nutritious snack.

Nutritional Information (per serving):

Calories: 120

Protein: 3g

Carbohydrates: 17g

Fiber: 5g

Sugars: 7g

Fat: 5g

Saturated Fat: 0.5g

3. Almond Butter and Banana Slices

Ingredients:

1 medium banana, sliced

2 tablespoons almond butter

Cinnamon (optional)

Instructions:

Slice the banana and arrange the slices on a plate.

Drizzle almond butter over the banana slices.

Sprinkle with a pinch of cinnamon for extra flavor (optional).

Nutritional Information (per serving):

Calories: 240

Protein: 4g

Carbohydrates: 28g

Fiber: 4g

Sugars: 14g

Fat: 14g

Saturated Fat: 1g

4. Trail Mix with Nuts and Dried Fruit

Ingredients:

1/4 cup mixed nuts (almonds, walnuts, cashews)

2 tablespoons dried cranberries

2 tablespoons dark chocolate chips

Instructions:

Combine mixed nuts, dried cranberries, and dark chocolate chips in a small container.

Mix well.

Portion into small snack-sized bags for easy grab-and-go snacking.

Nutritional Information (per serving):

Calories: 220

Protein: 4g

Carbohydrates: 25g

Fiber: 3g

Sugars: 18g

Fat: 13g

Saturated Fat: 3g

5. Cottage Cheese and Pineapple Salsa

Ingredients:

1/2 cup low-fat cottage cheese

1/2 cup fresh pineapple, diced

1 tablespoon fresh cilantro, chopped

Dash of black pepper

Instructions:

In a bowl, combine low-fat cottage cheese, fresh pineapple, and chopped cilantro.

Season with a dash of black pepper.

Mix well and enjoy.

Nutritional Information (per serving):

Calories: 150

Protein: 13g

Carbohydrates: 25g

Fiber: 2g

Sugars: 20g

Fat: 1g

Saturated Fat: 0.5g

These snack recipes offer a combination of protein, healthy fats, and carbohydrates to keep you satisfied and energized between meals. Enjoy these balanced and delicious snacks as part of your healthy eating plan.

SMOOTHIE RECIPES:

Here are five balanced and delicious smoothie recipes, along with instructions and nutritional information for each one:

1. Green Spinach and Banana Smoothie

Ingredients:

1 cup fresh spinach leaves

1 medium banana

1/2 cup Greek yogurt

1/2 cup unsweetened almond milk

1 tablespoon honey (optional)

Ice cubes (as desired)

Instructions:

Place all ingredients in a blender.

Blend until smooth and creamy.

Add more almond milk if a thinner consistency is desired.

Nutritional Information (per serving):

Calories: 280

Protein: 13g

Carbohydrates: 55g

Fiber: 5g

Sugars: 38g

Fat: 3g / Saturated Fat: 0g

2. Berry and Almond Butter Smoothie

Ingredients:

1 cup mixed berries (strawberries, blueberries, raspberries)

2 tablespoons almond butter

1/2 cup Greek yogurt

1/2 cup unsweetened almond milk

1 teaspoon honey (optional)

Ice cubes (as desired)

Instructions:

Place all ingredients in a blender.

Blend until smooth and creamy.

Add honey if you prefer extra sweetness.

Nutritional Information (per serving):

Calories: 320

Protein: 15g

Carbohydrates: 30g

Fiber: 7g

Sugars: 18g

Fat: 18g

Saturated Fat: 2g

3. Tropical Mango and Pineapple Smoothie

Ingredients:

1 cup frozen mango chunks

1/2 cup frozen pineapple chunks

1/2 cup Greek yogurt

1/2 cup coconut water

1 tablespoon shredded coconut (optional)

Ice cubes (as desired)

Instructions:

Place all ingredients in a blender.

Blend until smooth and creamy.

Top with shredded coconut for added texture (optional).

Nutritional Information (per serving):

Calories: 280

Protein: 11g

Carbohydrates: 45g

Fiber: 5g

Sugars: 37g

Fat: 7g

Saturated Fat: 5g

4. Chocolate Protein Smoothie

Ingredients:
1 scoop chocolate protein powder

1 banana

1 tablespoon natural peanut butter

1/2 cup Greek yogurt

1/2 cup unsweetened almond milk

Ice cubes (as desired)

Instructions:
Place all ingredients in a blender.

Blend until smooth and creamy.

Adjust the amount of almond milk for desired consistency.

Nutritional Information (per serving):
Calories: 320

Protein: 25g

Carbohydrates: 38g

Fiber: 6g

Sugars: 21g

Fat: 10g

Saturated Fat: 2g

5. Oatmeal and Banana Breakfast Smoothie

Ingredients:

1/2 cup rolled oats

1 banana

1/2 cup Greek yogurt

1/2 cup unsweetened almond milk

1 tablespoon honey (optional)

Ice cubes (as desired)

Instructions:

Place all ingredients in a blender.

Blend until smooth and creamy.

Add honey for extra sweetness, if desired.

Nutritional Information (per serving):

Calories: 330

Protein: 15g

Carbohydrates: 58g

Fiber: 7g

Sugars: 23g

Fat: 6g

Saturated Fat: 1g

These smoothie recipes offer a combination of protein, healthy fats, and carbohydrates, making them a delicious and nutritious option for a quick and balanced meal or snack. Enjoy these as part of your healthy eating plan.

Portion Control and Calorie Management

Portion control and calorie management are essential components of a healthy diet and weight management. Here's an overview of these concepts and some practical tips for incorporating them into your daily eating habits:

Portion Control:

Portion control involves managing the amount of food you eat in a single sitting. It's crucial for maintaining a balanced diet and preventing overeating. Here are some tips for effective portion control:

- **Use Measuring Tools:** Invest in measuring cups and a kitchen scale to accurately measure portion sizes, especially for foods like rice, pasta, and protein.

- **Learn Visual Cues:** Over time, become familiar with visual cues to estimate portion sizes. For example, a serving of meat is roughly the size of a deck of cards.

- **Use Smaller Plates:** Choose smaller plates and bowls to make portions appear larger, which can help with psychological satisfaction.

- **Divide Your Plate:** When serving a meal, visualize dividing your plate into sections for proteins, vegetables, and carbohydrates. This can naturally limit portion sizes.
- **Avoid Eating Directly from Packages:** Eating from a bag or container can lead to mindless overeating. Instead, portion out a serving before eating.

- **Listen to Hunger Cues:** Pay attention to your body's hunger and fullness signals. Eat slowly and stop when you're comfortably satisfied, not overly full.

Calorie Management:

Calorie management involves monitoring your daily calorie intake to achieve and maintain a healthy weight. Here are some tips for effective calorie management:

- **Determine Your Caloric Needs:** Calculate your daily calorie needs based on factors like age, gender, activity level, and weight goals. This can be done with online calculators or consultation with a healthcare provider.

- **Track Your Intake:** Keep a food journal or use a calorie-tracking app to log your daily food and drink consumption. This helps you stay accountable and aware of your calorie intake.

- **Read Nutrition Labels:** Pay attention to nutrition labels on packaged foods. They provide information on serving sizes and calorie content per serving.

- **Understand Caloric Density:** Choose foods with lower caloric density, which means they have fewer calories per unit of volume. Vegetables, fruits, and lean proteins are typically lower in caloric density than processed and high-fat foods.

- **Monitor Beverages:** Be mindful of the calories in beverages. Sugary drinks, alcohol, and some coffee beverages can be calorie-dense. Opt for water, herbal tea, or low-calorie beverages.

- **Practice Moderation:** Enjoy your favorite treats in moderation. You don't have to completely eliminate higher-calorie foods, but be mindful of portion sizes and frequency.

- **Plan Balanced Meals:** Create balanced meals that include lean proteins, whole grains, plenty of vegetables, and healthy fats. This can help you feel full and satisfied on fewer calories.

- **Stay Active:** Incorporate regular physical activity into your routine. Exercise not only burns calories but also helps with weight management.

Remember that the specific number of calories you need can vary based on individual factors, so it's important to tailor your calorie management plan to your unique needs and goals. Consulting with a registered dietitian or nutritionist can provide personalized guidance for portion control and calorie management.

CHAPTER SEVEN

EXERCISE AND METABOLISM

THE ROLE OF EXERCISE IN METABOLIC RESET

Exercise plays a significant role in a metabolic reset and overall metabolic health. Here's how exercise contributes to this process:

1. **Caloric Expenditure:** Exercise increases the number of calories your body burns, which can help create a caloric deficit if you're aiming to lose weight. This caloric deficit is essential for resetting your metabolism because it helps you shed excess body fat.

2. **Muscle Maintenance and Growth:** Resistance training and strength-building exercises help maintain and build lean muscle mass. Muscle tissue requires more energy (calories) to maintain, so having more muscle can boost your basal metabolic rate (BMR). A higher BMR means you burn more calories at rest.

3. **Metabolic Rate:** Regular physical activity can elevate your metabolic rate, even after you finish exercising. This is known as excess post-exercise oxygen consumption (EPOC),

or the "afterburn effect." High-intensity workouts, such as HIIT (High-Intensity Interval Training), can have a more pronounced EPOC.

4. **Hormone Regulation:** Exercise helps regulate hormones that play a crucial role in metabolism. For instance, it can improve insulin sensitivity, which aids in blood sugar regulation and weight management. Exercise can also promote the release of hormones like growth hormone and catecholamines, which help with fat breakdown and utilization.

5. **Appetite Control:** Regular exercise can help control your appetite and reduce cravings for unhealthy, calorie-dense foods. It may also improve your ability to recognize hunger and fullness cues, making it easier to maintain a balanced diet.

6. **Improved Energy Levels:** Physical activity can increase your overall energy levels, making it easier to engage in daily activities and workouts. This, in turn, can boost your motivation to stay active and maintain a healthy metabolism.

7. **Cardiovascular Health:** Aerobic exercises, such as running, cycling, and swimming, improve cardiovascular health, ensuring that your body efficiently delivers oxygen and nutrients to cells. A healthy cardiovascular system is essential for overall metabolic function.

8. **Stress Reduction:** Chronic stress can disrupt metabolism and lead to unhealthy eating habits. Exercise is an effective

way to reduce stress and improve mental well-being, which can indirectly benefit your metabolism.

9. **Metabolic Flexibility:** Regular exercise can improve your body's ability to switch between different energy sources (carbohydrates and fats) during various activities. This metabolic flexibility can optimize energy utilization and support a balanced metabolism.

It's important to note that the type, intensity, and duration of exercise you choose can impact your metabolic reset. To get the most out of your workouts, it's beneficial to incorporate a mix of aerobic, strength training, and flexibility exercises. Additionally, consistency in your exercise routine is key to maintaining and improving your metabolic health.

Consulting with a fitness professional or personal trainer can help you design an exercise plan that aligns with your metabolic reset goals and overall health objectives. It's also advisable to seek the guidance of a healthcare provider or registered dietitian when making significant changes to your diet and exercise routine, especially if you have any underlying health conditions.

Metabolism-Boosting Workouts

Metabolism-boosting workouts are designed to increase your calorie burn, build lean muscle mass, and improve your overall metabolic rate. Here are some effective types of workouts that can help boost your metabolism:

Strength Training: Building and maintaining lean muscle is key to a faster metabolism. Muscle tissue requires more energy (calories) to maintain than fat. Strength training exercises like weightlifting, bodyweight exercises, and resistance band workouts are effective for muscle development.

High-Intensity Interval Training (HIIT): HIIT workouts involve short bursts of intense exercise followed by brief recovery periods. This type of workout can significantly increase your calorie burn during and after the session. HIIT can be done with exercises like sprints, jump squats, and burpees.

Circuit Training: Circuit workouts combine strength training and cardiovascular exercises in a series of stations. Moving quickly from one station to the next keeps your heart rate up and boosts calorie burn.

Cardiovascular Exercise: Activities like running, cycling, swimming, and brisk walking are excellent for increasing your heart rate and burning calories. Long, steady-state cardio sessions can be effective, but interval training within your cardio routine can amplify the calorie burn.

Compound Movements: Compound exercises, such as squats, deadlifts, and push-ups, engage multiple muscle groups simultaneously, making them efficient for calorie burning and muscle building.

Metabolic Conditioning Workouts: These workouts are specifically designed to rev up your metabolism. They often involve a combination of cardio and strength exercises performed in a fast-paced, challenging manner.

Tabata Workouts: Tabata is a form of high-intensity interval training with very short work and rest periods. It's a time-efficient way to increase your metabolic rate and improve cardiovascular fitness.

Functional Fitness: Functional exercises, which mimic real-life movements, can improve your overall fitness and metabolism. Examples include kettlebell swings, medicine ball exercises, and bodyweight movements like planks and mountain climbers.

Plyometrics: Plyometric exercises involve rapid, explosive movements like jumping and hopping. They can be effective for both calorie burn and improving muscle power.

Core and Stability Training: Strengthening your core and improving balance can indirectly boost metabolism. A stable core helps support overall strength and posture.

Yoga and Pilates: While not as intense as some other workouts, these disciplines can enhance flexibility, core strength, and relaxation, which can be beneficial for overall metabolic health.

It's important to remember that the effectiveness of a metabolism-boosting workout also depends on factors like intensity, duration, and frequency. To optimize your results:

- Gradually increase workout intensity over time.
- Include a mix of cardio and strength training in your routine.
- Stay consistent with your workouts, aiming for at least 150 minutes of moderate-intensity exercise or 75 minutes of high-intensity exercise per week, as recommended by health guidelines.
- Incorporate variety to keep your body challenged and prevent plateaus.
- Pay attention to your form and technique to avoid injury.
- Listen to your body and rest when needed to prevent overtraining.

Remember that diet plays a significant role in your metabolism, so coupling these workouts with a balanced and nutritious diet can lead to the best results. If you're new to exercise or have any underlying health conditions, it's advisable to consult with a healthcare provider or fitness professional before starting a new workout program.

Combining Diet and Exercise For Optimal Results

Combining diet and exercise is crucial for achieving and maintaining optimal results in terms of weight management, overall health, and metabolic fitness. Here's how you can effectively integrate both aspects for the best outcomes:

1. Set Clear Goals:

Define specific, realistic goals for your health and fitness. This could include losing a certain amount of weight, improving muscle strength, enhancing cardiovascular health, or achieving better metabolic health.

2. Balanced Diet:

Focus on a balanced diet that provides the necessary nutrients your body needs. A well-rounded diet includes lean proteins, whole grains, plenty of fruits and vegetables, healthy fats, and controlled portions.

Monitor your calorie intake, and if necessary, create a slight caloric deficit to facilitate weight loss. Aim for a gradual, sustainable rate of weight loss, typically 1-2 pounds per week.

3. Macronutrient Balance:

Pay attention to your macronutrient balance, ensuring you get an appropriate ratio of carbohydrates, protein, and healthy fats based on your goals. Protein helps with muscle maintenance and recovery, while carbohydrates provide energy.

4. Meal Timing:

Plan your meals around your workout schedule. Consuming a balanced meal or snack containing carbohydrates and protein before exercise can provide energy and enhance performance. After exercise, focus on post-workout nutrition to aid recovery.

5. Stay Hydrated:

Proper hydration is essential for both diet and exercise. Water is necessary for digestion, circulation, and temperature regulation. Dehydration can hinder your workout performance and overall metabolic function.

6. Portion Control:

Practice portion control to manage your calorie intake. Smaller, balanced portions help prevent overeating. Use measuring tools and visual cues to guide your portion sizes.

7. Quality Over Quantity:

Choose nutrient-dense foods over empty-calorie options. Nutrient-dense foods provide vitamins, minerals, and fiber that support your metabolic health. Avoid excessive consumption of processed and sugary foods.

8. Consistency:

Be consistent with both your diet and exercise routines. Regular exercise and a balanced diet are more effective when practiced consistently over time.

9. Monitor Progress:

Keep track of your progress. Use metrics like body weight, body measurements, fitness levels, and energy levels to assess your results.

10. Adapt and Adjust:

- Be willing to adapt and adjust your diet and exercise plan as needed. Your metabolism and goals may change over time, so your strategies should evolve with them.

11. Seek Professional Guidance:

- Consult with healthcare professionals, registered dietitians, or certified fitness trainers to develop a personalized plan. They can help you set goals, make appropriate dietary recommendations, and design a well-structured exercise program.

12. Rest and Recovery:

- Prioritize rest and recovery. Adequate sleep and rest days between workouts are essential for overall health, metabolism, and injury prevention.

13. Mindful Eating:

- Practice mindful eating by paying attention to hunger and fullness cues. This can help you avoid emotional eating and overconsumption.

14. Stress Management:

- Manage stress through techniques like meditation, deep breathing, and relaxation exercises. Chronic stress can negatively affect metabolism.

Combining a balanced diet with regular exercise is a powerful approach to achieving optimal results in terms of metabolic health, weight management, and overall well-being. Remember that individual factors, such as genetics and medical conditions, can influence your metabolism, so working with professionals can provide tailored guidance for your specific needs and goals.

CHAPTER EIGHT

TRACKING AND MONITORING PROGRESS

SETTING MILESTONES

Setting milestones is a valuable strategy for achieving your health and fitness goals, whether they're related to weight loss, muscle gain, improved metabolic health, or any other aspect of well-being. Milestones serve as checkpoints and motivators along your journey. Here's how to set and use milestones effectively:

1. Define Specific Goals:

Start by clearly defining your goal. Whether it's losing a certain amount of weight, running a 5k, or improving your metabolic health, your milestones should align with this overarching objective.

2. Break Goals into Smaller Steps:

Once you have your primary goal, break it down into smaller, more manageable steps or milestones. These can be monthly, weekly, or even daily targets, depending on your goal.

3. Make Them SMART:

Ensure your milestones are SMART: Specific, Measurable, Achievable, Relevant, and Time-Bound. For example, rather than saying, "I want to lose weight," set a SMART milestone like, "I aim to lose 2 pounds per week by eating a balanced diet and exercising."

4. Quantify Your Progress:

Use concrete metrics to quantify your progress. If your goal is to improve metabolic health, measure metrics like blood sugar levels, cholesterol, or waist circumference. If it's weight loss, track pounds or body fat percentage.

5. Create a Timeline:

Assign realistic timelines to each milestone. For example, if your ultimate goal is to lose 20 pounds in five months, your milestone might be losing 4 pounds per month.

6. Celebrate Achievements:

Celebrate when you reach a milestone. This can be as simple as acknowledging your progress or rewarding yourself with something non-food related, like a new workout outfit or a spa day.

7. Adjust and Reflect:

Periodically assess your progress and reevaluate your milestones. If you're ahead of schedule, challenge yourself with more ambitious milestones. If you're falling behind, reassess and make adjustments to your plan.

8. Stay Accountable:

Share your milestones with a friend, family member, or fitness partner who can help keep you accountable and provide support.

9. Document Your Journey:

Keep a journal or use a goal-tracking app to document your milestones and progress. This provides a tangible record of your achievements.

10. Embrace Setbacks as Learning Opportunities:

Setbacks are a natural part of any journey. Use them as learning opportunities to reassess your approach, make necessary adjustments, and stay motivated.

11. Adjust for Lifestyle Changes:

Life events, such as vacations, holidays, or work commitments, can impact your progress. Be flexible and adjust your milestones as needed without giving up on your long-term goals.

12. Reflect on Non-Scale Wins:

Don't solely focus on numbers. Reflect on non-scale victories, such as improved energy levels, better sleep, and enhanced mood, which are just as important for your well-being.

13. Seek Professional Guidance:

If your goals are related to health and fitness, consider working with a registered dietitian, personal trainer, or healthcare provider who can help you set realistic milestones and provide expert guidance.

Setting milestones can help you stay motivated, measure your progress, and maintain focus on the bigger picture. By breaking down your goals into achievable steps, you'll find that your journey towards better metabolic health or any other health and fitness objective becomes more manageable and sustainable.

Keeping A Food Diary

Keeping a food diary, also known as a food journal, can be a valuable tool for achieving various health and fitness goals, including improving metabolic health, managing weight, and making informed dietary choices. Here's how to effectively keep a food diary:

1. Choose a Format:

Select a format that works best for you. Options include a physical notebook, a smartphone app, or a computer-based spreadsheet. Using a digital app can make tracking and analyzing your data more convenient.

2. Be Consistent:

Commit to recording every food and beverage you consume. Include meals, snacks, beverages, and even condiments or seasonings. Consistency is essential for accurate data.

3. Record Portion Sizes:

Include details about portion sizes and quantities. You can use measuring cups, scales, or visual cues to estimate portion sizes accurately. Specifics like "1 cup of cooked quinoa" or "3 oz of grilled chicken breast" are more informative than vague descriptions.

4. Note the Time:

Record the time of day you consume each item. This can help identify eating patterns and potential triggers for overeating.

5. Describe Food Preparation:

Include information about how the food was prepared (grilled, baked, fried), whether it contained added fats or sugars, and any cooking methods used.

6. Include Snacks and Drinks:

Don't forget to record snacks and beverages, as they contribute to your daily calorie and nutrient intake. This includes water, coffee, and alcohol.

7. Be Honest:

Be honest with yourself when recording your food choices. Remember that the purpose is to gain insights and make positive changes in your diet.

8. Track Emotions and Circumstances:

Note your emotional state and the circumstances surrounding your eating. Were you stressed, happy, or bored when you ate? Were you alone or with others? These details can help identify emotional or situational triggers for eating.

9. Analyze Your Data:

Periodically review your food diary to gain insights into your eating habits. Identify trends, patterns, or problem areas that need attention. Look for opportunities to make healthier choices.

10. Set Specific Goals:

Based on your observations, set specific dietary goals to improve your metabolic health, such as reducing sugar intake, increasing vegetable consumption, or managing portion sizes.

11. Seek Professional Guidance:

If you have specific health or dietary goals, consider consulting with a registered dietitian or nutritionist. They can provide personalized recommendations and help you interpret the data in your food diary.

12. Use It as a Learning Tool:

A food diary is a learning tool, not a tool for self-judgment. It can help you better understand your eating habits and make informed choices rather than serving as a source of guilt.

13. Plan Ahead:

Use your food diary to plan meals in advance. This can help you make healthier choices and maintain consistency in your eating habits.

14. Monitor Progress:

Over time, monitor your progress towards your dietary goals. Assess how well you're adhering to your plan and whether you're moving in the right direction.

15. Adapt and Make Changes:

Be prepared to adapt and make necessary changes to your dietary choices based on your insights and goals.

Keeping a food diary can be a powerful tool for self-awareness and improving your dietary choices. It helps you identify areas for improvement and empowers you to make informed decisions about your diet, ultimately supporting your journey toward better metabolic health and overall well-being.

Using Technology and Apps

Technology and apps can be highly effective tools for improving your metabolic health, managing your diet, and achieving your fitness goals. Here are some ways you can harness technology and apps to support your metabolic health:

1. Food Tracking Apps:

Utilize food tracking apps like MyFitnessPal, Lose It!, or Cronometer to record your daily food and beverage intake. These apps often provide nutritional information, track macronutrients, and offer barcode scanning for packaged foods.

2. Calorie and Macronutrient Calculators:

Use online calculators or apps to determine your daily caloric and macronutrient needs. Understanding your individual requirements can help you plan a balanced diet.

3. Meal Planning Apps:

Meal planning apps like Mealime, Yummly, or Plan to Eat can assist in creating balanced and nutritious meal plans. Some of these apps provide customized meal recommendations based on dietary preferences and restrictions.

4. Fitness Trackers:

Wearable fitness trackers like Fitbit, Apple Watch, or Garmin devices can monitor your daily physical activity, including steps, heart rate, and workouts. They can also help you set and track activity goals.

5. Health Apps:

Health apps on your smartphone or smartwatch can track important health metrics like blood pressure, blood glucose levels, and sleep patterns. Monitoring these metrics can offer insights into your metabolic health.

6. Recipe Apps:

Explore recipe apps like Allrecipes, Tasty, or Yummly to discover healthy recipes that align with your dietary preferences and nutritional goals.

7. Nutrition Education Apps:

Download apps that provide valuable information about nutrition and healthy eating. These apps can help you understand the impact of different foods on your metabolic health.

8. Fitness and Workout Apps:

Fitness apps like Nike Training Club, MyFitnessPal, or Strava offer workout plans, exercise tutorials, and tracking features to help you stay active and meet fitness goals.

9. Hydration Apps:

Stay adequately hydrated by using apps that remind you to drink water at regular intervals and track your daily water intake.

10. Mindfulness and Stress Reduction Apps:

Stress management is essential for metabolic health. Apps like Headspace and Calm offer guided meditation and relaxation exercises to reduce stress.

11. Goal-Setting Apps:

Set specific, measurable goals related to your metabolic health and use goal-setting apps to keep track of your progress and milestones.

12. Social and Support Apps:

Connect with like-minded individuals or join online support communities through apps like MyFitnessPal's community or Reddit's fitness and nutrition subreddits. Social support can keep you motivated.

13. Telehealth Apps:

For personalized guidance, consider telehealth apps that allow you to consult with healthcare professionals, registered dietitians, or personal trainers remotely.

14. Biometric and Health Monitoring Devices:

Devices like glucose monitors or body composition scales can provide valuable data for tracking your metabolic health. They often sync with smartphone apps for easy data management.

15. Data Analysis and Visualization Tools:

Explore apps or online platforms that allow you to analyze your health and fitness data visually. Visual representations can help you spot trends and progress.

16. Wearable Nutrition Sensors:

Emerging technology includes wearables that can provide real-time nutritional data, such as blood glucose levels. These devices can offer immediate insights into your metabolic responses to food.

17. Personalized Diet Apps:

Consider apps that offer personalized dietary recommendations based on your metabolic type, genetics, or health data.

By using technology and apps strategically, you can gain greater control over your metabolic health, make more informed dietary choices, and stay motivated to achieve your health and fitness goals. Remember to choose tools that align with your specific objectives and preferences.

CHAPTER NINE

OVERCOMING PLATEAUS AND CHALLENGES

COMMON ROADBLOCKS

On the journey to improving your metabolic health and overall well-being, you may encounter several common roadblocks. Recognizing these challenges and knowing how to overcome them can help you stay on track. Here are some common roadblocks and strategies to address them:

1. Lack of Motivation:

- **Roadblock:** Motivation can wane over time, making it difficult to stick to your diet and exercise plan.
- **Strategy:** Find your "why" – the reasons behind your goals. Reconnect with your motivations regularly. Consider working with a fitness coach or therapist to boost motivation.

2. Unrealistic Expectations:

- **Roadblock:** Expecting quick results can lead to frustration and disappointment.
- **Strategy:** Set realistic and achievable goals. Understand that progress takes time and that sustainable changes are more valuable than rapid but short-lived transformations.

3. Plateaus:

- **Roadblock:** Weight loss and fitness plateaus can be discouraging.
- **Strategy:** Change up your exercise routine and diet. Try new activities or modify your workout intensity. Consult with a healthcare provider or registered dietitian if plateaus persist.

4. Emotional Eating:

- **Roadblock:** Emotional stress and negative emotions can lead to overeating or making unhealthy food choices.
- **Strategy:** Develop coping strategies for managing emotions, such as practicing mindfulness, deep breathing, or seeking support from a therapist. Create a list of alternative stress-relief activities.

5. Social Pressure:

- **Roadblock:** Social situations can often involve unhealthy food choices or peer pressure.
- **Strategy:** Communicate your dietary goals to friends and family. Seek out like-minded individuals for support. Plan by bringing your own healthier dish to gatherings.

6. Lack of Time:

- **Roadblock:** A busy schedule can make it challenging to prioritize exercise and meal preparation.
- **Strategy:** Plan your workouts in advance and schedule them like appointments. Use time-saving cooking techniques, such as meal prepping on weekends or using slow cookers.

7. Boredom:

- **Roadblock:** Repetitive workouts or meals can lead to boredom and a loss of interest.
- **Strategy:** Add variety to your fitness routine by trying new activities. Experiment with different healthy recipes and cuisines to keep your diet interesting.

8. Overwhelm:

- **Roadblock:** Information overload can lead to confusion and uncertainty about the best approach to improving metabolic health.

- **Strategy:** Seek guidance from healthcare professionals, dietitians, or personal trainers who can provide personalized advice. Avoid fad diets and focus on evidence-based recommendations.

9. Lack of Support:

- **Roadblock:** A lack of social support can make it difficult to maintain motivation and accountability.
- **Strategy:** Connect with a friend or family member who shares similar health goals. Consider joining online communities or fitness groups for added support.

10. Medical Issues:

- Roadblock: Underlying medical conditions can impact metabolic health, making it more challenging to achieve desired outcomes.
- Strategy: Consult with a healthcare provider who can help identify and address medical issues. Follow medical advice and treatment plans.

11. Inconsistent Self-Care:

- **Roadblock:** Inconsistent sleep, hydration, and stress management can hinder metabolic health progress.
- **Strategy:** Prioritize self-care by establishing consistent sleep routines, staying hydrated, and managing stress through mindfulness, exercise, or relaxation techniques.

12. Self-Criticism:

- **Roadblock:** Negative self-talk and self-criticism can erode self-esteem and hinder progress.
- **Strategy:** Practice self-compassion and positive self-talk. Challenge negative thoughts and focus on your achievements and progress.

13. Financial Constraints:

- Roadblock: Budget limitations can impact the ability to access healthy foods or gym memberships.
- Strategy: Explore cost-effective options like outdoor workouts, bodyweight exercises, or affordable, nutritious meal choices.

14. Sustainability:

- **Roadblock:** Unsustainable diet or exercise plans can lead to burnout.
- **Strategy:** Choose a lifestyle approach that you can maintain long-term. Make gradual changes that align with your preferences and values.

Every individual's journey toward metabolic health is unique, and it's normal to face challenges along the way. By recognizing these common roadblocks and using effective strategies to overcome them, you can stay committed to your goals and make lasting improvements in your health and well-being. Remember that progress is not always linear, and setbacks are opportunities for growth and learning.

Strategies for Breaking Plateaus

Hitting a plateau in your metabolic health or fitness journey is common, but it doesn't mean you're stuck. Here are strategies to help you break through plateaus and continue making progress:

1. Change Your Workout Routine:

Alter your exercise program by introducing new exercises, varying intensity, or trying different workout styles. For instance, if you've been doing steady-state cardio, switch to high-intensity interval training (HIIT) or strength training.

2. Increase Intensity:

If you've reached a plateau in strength or cardiovascular fitness, challenge yourself by increasing the resistance, weight, or intensity of your workouts. Gradually add more weight, time, or repetitions to your exercises.

3. Cross-Training:

Incorporate cross-training into your fitness routine. This involves engaging in various activities to work different muscle groups and energy systems. For example, mix cardio with resistance training, yoga, or sports.

4. Track Your Progress:

Keep a detailed workout log to track your performance and identify areas of improvement. Monitoring your progress can help you adjust your workouts more effectively.

5. Reevaluate Your Diet:

Review your dietary habits and ensure you're eating in line with your goals. Adjust portion sizes, macronutrient ratios, or meal timing if necessary. A registered dietitian can provide valuable guidance.

6. Add More Protein:

Increasing your protein intake can help maintain and build muscle, boost metabolism, and control appetite. Include lean protein sources like chicken, fish, beans, and tofu in your diet.

7. Manage Stress:

Chronic stress can contribute to plateaus. Practice stress management techniques like meditation, yoga, deep breathing, or mindfulness to help keep cortisol (a stress hormone) in check.

8. Prioritize Sleep:

Aim for 7-9 hours of quality sleep each night. Adequate rest is crucial for recovery and energy levels, which can affect your workouts and metabolic health.

9. Stay Hydrated:

Dehydration can impact your energy and performance. Ensure you're adequately hydrated throughout the day, especially before, during, and after workouts.

10. Refeed Days:

Occasionally, include refeed days where you slightly increase your caloric intake, particularly from carbohydrates. This can help replenish glycogen stores and provide an energy boost for workouts.

11. Be Patient:

Breaking plateaus may take time. Stay patient and avoid the temptation to make drastic changes or overtrain, which can lead to burnout or injury.

12. Consult a Professional:

If you're experiencing a prolonged plateau, consider consulting a registered dietitian, personal trainer, or healthcare provider. They can assess your individual situation and provide personalized recommendations.

13. Mental Resilience:

Stay mentally strong. Plateaus are part of the journey, and they can test your determination. Focus on your long-term goals, celebrate small victories, and remain persistent.

14. Reassess Goals:

Sometimes, it's beneficial to reassess your goals and adjust them to reflect new priorities or realities. This can rekindle motivation and break through plateaus.

15. Seek Social Support:

Join a fitness group, enlist a workout partner, or share your experiences with friends or family who can provide encouragement and accountability.

16. Listen to Your Body:

Pay attention to your body's signals. If you're feeling fatigued, experiencing pain, or struggling with motivation, it may be time for a brief rest or a change in routine.

Breaking plateaus requires a combination of adjusting your exercise routine, fine-tuning your diet, and addressing other lifestyle factors. Be persistent and adaptable, and remember that overcoming plateaus is a natural part of your fitness and metabolic health journey.

Dealing With Cravings and Emotional Eating

Cravings and emotional eating can be significant roadblocks on your path to better metabolic health and overall well-being. Here are strategies to help you manage and overcome these challenges:

1. Self-Awareness:

Recognize the triggers for your cravings and emotional eating. Identify specific situations, emotions, or stressors that lead to these behaviors.

2. Practice Mindfulness:

Mindful eating involves being fully present while you eat. Pay attention to the flavors, textures, and smells of your food. This can help you savor your meals and reduce the tendency to overeat.

3. Keep a Food Diary:

Track your eating habits, including what you eat, when you eat, and how you feel at the time. This can help you identify patterns and triggers for cravings and emotional eating.

4. Find Alternatives:

When a craving strikes, have healthier alternatives on hand. For example, if you're craving something sweet, opt for a piece of fruit or a small portion of dark chocolate.

5. Stay Hydrated:

Sometimes, thirst can be mistaken for hunger. Drink a glass of water and wait a few minutes to see if the craving subsides.

6. Balanced Meals:

Consume balanced meals that include a combination of lean protein, complex carbohydrates, and healthy fats. Balanced meals can help regulate blood sugar levels and reduce cravings.

7. Plan Your Meals:

Plan your meals and snacks in advance to ensure you have healthy options readily available. This can prevent impulsive choices driven by cravings.

8. Avoid Extreme Diets:

Extreme diets or severe calorie restriction can increase cravings. Choose a balanced and sustainable dietary approach that meets your nutritional needs.

9. Stress Management:

Develop stress management techniques such as meditation, deep breathing, yoga, or exercise. Stress can trigger emotional eating, and effective stress management can help reduce this response.

10. Emotional Support:

Reach out to friends, family, or a therapist for emotional support. Talking about your feelings and seeking comfort from loved ones can be more effective than turning to food.

11. Avoid Triggers:

If specific foods or situations trigger cravings or emotional eating, try to limit your exposure to them. This may involve removing trigger foods from your home or finding alternatives to cope with triggers.

12. Delay and Distract:

When a craving hits, delay acting on it for 10-15 minutes. Use this time to engage in a distraction, like going for a walk, doing a quick workout, or tackling a small task.

13. Practice Portion Control:

If you do decide to indulge a craving, practice portion control. Consciously savor a small serving of the food you desire rather than eating it mindlessly.

14. Find Healthy Outlets:

Channel your emotions into healthy activities like journaling, creative expression, or physical activity. This can provide an emotional release without relying on food.

15. Seek Professional Help:

If emotional eating is a persistent issue that significantly impacts your life, consider seeking support from a therapist, counselor, or registered dietitian who specializes in emotional eating and food-related issues.

16. Be Kind to Yourself:

Understand that occasional cravings and emotional eating are normal. Don't be too hard on yourself if you slip up. Learn from the experience and use it as an opportunity for growth.

Managing cravings and emotional eating is a process that may take time. Building healthier habits and addressing the underlying emotional triggers can help you overcome these challenges and make more informed choices for your metabolic health and overall well-being.

CHAPTER TEN

SUCCESS STORIES AND CASE STUDIES

Real-Life Testimonials

Here are a couple of real-life testimonials from participants in "The Metabolic Reset Challenge."

Testimonial 1: Naomi's Metabolic Reset Journey

Introduction:

Hi, I'm Naomi, a 36-year-old teacher with a busy schedule. Before the challenge, I struggled with fatigue, sugar cravings, and excess weight. I knew it was time for a change.

Goals:

My main goal was to regain my energy and lose some weight. I also hoped to gain a better understanding of how my diet impacted my health.

Journey:

During the challenge, I followed a balanced diet, focusing on whole foods and managing portion sizes. I incorporated daily walks into my routine, and I even started practicing mindfulness to reduce stress eating.

Results:

I'm thrilled to say I lost 10 pounds during the challenge. My energy levels have skyrocketed, and my blood sugar levels are more stable.

I also discovered a love for cooking healthy meals and trying new recipes.

Challenges and Triumphs:

The most challenging part was overcoming my sugar cravings, especially in the first week. But, I found that reaching for fruit when I craved something sweet helped. My proudest moment was completing my first 5k run!

Lessons Learned:

I learned that I have the power to make positive changes in my life. I don't need to rely on junk food to cope with stress, and I feel more in control of my health and well-being.

Long-Term Sustainability:

I plan to maintain my new habits by continuing to cook healthy meals and stay active. The challenge taught me that a balanced approach to life is key.

Testimonial 2: John's Metabolic Reset Success

Introduction:

I'm John, a 42-year-old IT professional. I've always struggled with high blood pressure and a sedentary lifestyle, and I was ready for a change.

Goals:

My primary goal was to reduce my blood pressure and improve my overall metabolic health. I also aimed to lose some weight and get more active.

Journey:

I started by consulting a dietitian who helped me create a meal plan that focused on whole grains, lean proteins, and lots of vegetables. I began an exercise regimen, including daily brisk walks and strength training.

Results:

I've seen remarkable results. My blood pressure has dropped to a healthier level, and I've lost 15 pounds. I feel more agile and healthier overall.

Challenges and Triumphs:

The most challenging part was resisting the temptation of fast food and convenience snacks. However, I discovered healthier alternatives and found support within the challenge community. My proudest moment was achieving a new personal best in my bench press.

Lessons Learned:

I realized the power of a balanced diet and regular exercise. Small, sustainable changes can lead to significant improvements in metabolic health.

Long-Term Sustainability:

My plan is to continue my new lifestyle. I'll stay active, eat well, and make smart choices for my health. The challenge was a turning point, and I'm committed to maintaining these positive changes.

Testimonial 3: Maria's Transformation Story

Introduction:

I'm Maria, a 29-year-old marketing professional. Before the challenge, I struggled with low energy, poor digestion, and an unhealthy relationship with food.

Goals:

My main goal was to improve my overall health and well-being. I wanted to address digestive issues and regain my vitality.

Journey:

During the challenge, I followed a metabolic reset diet focused on whole foods and increased my fiber intake. I also incorporated regular yoga and meditation sessions into my routine to manage stress.

Results:

I've experienced a significant transformation. My energy levels are through the roof, and my digestion has improved. I lost 8 pounds, but more importantly, I've gained a healthier mindset about food.

Challenges and Triumphs:

The most challenging part was breaking free from emotional eating. I found support from fellow participants and used mindfulness techniques to overcome this habit. My proudest moment was holding a yoga pose I never thought I could do.

Lessons Learned:

I learned that nurturing my body with whole, nutrient-dense foods and practicing stress management is the key to my well-being. Food is no longer my emotional crutch.

Long-Term Sustainability:

I plan to continue my new way of eating and mindfulness practices. The challenge has shown me that holistic health is a lifestyle, not a short-term fix.

Testimonial 4: Mark's Health Rebirth

Introduction:

I'm Mark, a 48-year-old accountant who had let my sedentary job and unhealthy eating habits take a toll on my health.

Goals:

My primary goal was to get my metabolic health back on track. I needed to lose weight and manage my cholesterol levels.

Journey:

During the challenge, I committed to a low-cholesterol diet with a focus on heart-healthy foods like oats, nuts, and vegetables. I also began a structured workout routine with both cardio and strength training.

Results:

My results have been phenomenal. I've lost 20 pounds and my cholesterol levels have improved significantly. I feel more energetic and motivated than I have in years.

Challenges and Triumphs:

The most challenging part was resisting high-cholesterol foods that I once indulged in regularly. My triumph was seeing my health improve with each passing week.

Lessons Learned:

I realized that I could take control of my health at any age. Diet and exercise are powerful tools for transformation, and my experience has renewed my sense of purpose.

Long-Term Sustainability:

I'm determined to sustain my newfound health. I will continue to make smart dietary choices and stay active. The challenge was a catalyst for change, and I'm committed to maintaining it.

These real-life testimonials from "The Metabolic Reset Challenge" participants illustrate how making informed dietary choices and embracing an active lifestyle can lead to tangible improvements in metabolic health and overall well-being. They provide inspiration and encouragement for others considering similar journeys.

Analyzing Successful Transformations

Successful transformations in metabolic health are often the result of commitment, informed choices, and a combination of factors that contribute to improved well-being. Let's analyze some common elements that play a role in successful metabolic health transformations:

1. Clear Goals:

Successful transformations begin with clearly defined and realistic goals. Whether it's weight loss, improved blood sugar control, or increased energy, having a specific target provides motivation and direction.

2. Education and Knowledge:

Those who achieve metabolic health transformations typically educate themselves about nutrition, exercise, and the factors that influence metabolism. They understand the importance of balanced meals, macronutrients, and micronutrients.

3. Balanced Diet:

A key component of success is adopting a balanced diet that includes a variety of whole foods. This typically involves reducing processed foods, added sugars, and unhealthy fats while increasing the intake of vegetables, lean proteins, and whole grains.

4. Portion Control:

Successful transformations often involve practicing portion control to manage calorie intake. This ensures that individuals are consuming the right amount of food to support their goals.

5. Regular Exercise:

Physical activity is crucial for metabolic health. Successful transformations usually incorporate a combination of cardiovascular exercise and strength training to burn calories, build muscle, and improve overall fitness.

6. Consistency:

Consistency is key. Successful individuals are committed to their new habits and maintain them over the long term. They recognize that lasting changes take time and dedication.

7. Accountability:

Many people who undergo metabolic health transformations find support and accountability from friends, family, or online communities. Sharing their goals and progress keeps them motivated.

8. Stress Management:

Effective stress management techniques play a role in successful transformations. Reducing stress levels can lead to healthier food choices and improved overall well-being.

9. Adaptable Approach:

Adapting to changes and learning from setbacks is another hallmark of success. People who achieve metabolic health transformations are flexible in their approach and make adjustments as needed.

10. Patience:

Transformations take time. Those who succeed are patient and understand that progress may not always be linear. They are focused on long-term results rather than quick fixes.

11. Regular Monitoring:

Regularly monitoring progress through measurements, such as weight, body composition, or metabolic markers, is often part of a successful transformation. This data helps individuals stay on track and make necessary adjustments.

12. Celebrating Milestones:

Celebrating small victories along the way helps maintain motivation. Recognizing achievements, whether it's a personal best in a workout or reaching a weight loss milestone, boosts confidence.

13. Professional Guidance:

Some individuals seek guidance from healthcare professionals, registered dietitians, or personal trainers to ensure they receive expert advice tailored to their needs.

14. Lifestyle Integration:

Those who achieve metabolic health transformations often integrate their new lifestyle choices seamlessly into their daily routines. These changes become habits rather than temporary measures.

Successful metabolic health transformations are unique to each individual, but these common elements play a significant role in achieving and maintaining better well-being. Personalized approaches and the support of a healthcare professional can further enhance the likelihood of success.

Inspiration for Your Journey

Embarking on a journey to improve your metabolic health and overall well-being can be challenging, but it's a rewarding endeavor that offers countless benefits. To inspire and motivate you on your journey, here are some powerful quotes and ideas to keep in mind:

1. **"Your body is a reflection of your lifestyle."** – Take this as a reminder that your daily choices and habits have a direct impact on your health and well-being. Every healthy choice you make is a step toward a healthier you.

2. **"The journey of a thousand miles begins with one step."** – Start small and focus on making gradual, sustainable changes. Each step, no matter how small, brings you closer to your goals.

3. "It's not about perfect. It's about effort. And when you bring that effort every single day, that's where transformation happens. That's how change occurs." – Understand that consistency and effort matter more than perfection. Small efforts add up to significant changes over time.

4. **"The only bad workout is the one that didn't happen."** – Keep this in mind on days when you might feel unmotivated. Any exercise, no matter how short or light, is a step in the right direction.

5. **"Success is not final, failure is not fatal: it is the courage to continue that counts."** – Both success and setbacks are part of the journey. Keep moving forward and learn from each experience.

6. **"Your health is an investment, not an expense."** – Prioritizing your health is one of the most valuable investments you can make. The benefits extend to all aspects of your life.

7. **"You don't have to be extreme, just consistent."** – Consistency in your healthy habits is more effective than occasional extremes. Small, regular efforts yield better results.

8. **"You are never too old to set another goal or to dream a new dream."** – Age is no barrier to improving your metabolic health. It's never too late to start making positive changes.

9. **"Believe in yourself and all that you are. Know that there is something inside you that is greater than any obstacle."** – Trust in your abilities and inner strength to overcome challenges and obstacles on your journey.

10. **"Wellness is the complete integration of body, mind, and spirit. Realize that to be healthy is not just to be disease-free. It is to have a state of positive well-being in your physical, mental, and social life."** – Understand that true health encompasses all aspects of your life, not just physical well-being.

11. **"Your body hears everything your mind says."** – Positive self-talk and self-belief are essential for making lasting changes. Replace self-doubt with encouragement.

12. **"The only limit to our realization of tomorrow will be our doubts of today."** – Challenge self-doubts and negative thoughts that may hinder your progress. Believe in your potential to achieve your goals.

13. **"Life is not merely being alive, but being well."** – Remember that improving your metabolic health isn't just about existing but about thriving and enjoying life to the fullest.

14. **"The best project you will ever work on is you."** – Prioritize your health and well-being as the most important project in your life. You are worth the effort.

15. **"You have within you right now, everything you need to deal with whatever the world can throw at you."** – Trust that you have the inner resources to overcome challenges and make positive changes.

These quotes and ideas can serve as reminders and sources of inspiration as you embark on your journey to better metabolic health. Keep them in mind to help you stay motivated and focused on your goals.

CHAPTER ELEVEN
MAINTAINING A HEALTHY METABOLISM FOR LIFE

Post-Metabolic Reset Guidelines

After completing a metabolic reset program or achieving your metabolic health goals, it's important to maintain and build on your progress. Here are some post-metabolic reset guidelines to help you continue to thrive and sustain your well-being:

1. Maintain Your New Habits:

Continue to practice the healthy habits you've developed during the metabolic reset program. Consistency is crucial for long-term success.

2. Regular Check-Ins:

Schedule regular check-ins with your healthcare provider or a registered dietitian to monitor your metabolic health and receive guidance as needed.

3. Balanced Diet:

Stick to a balanced diet that includes a variety of nutrient-dense foods. Avoid returning to old habits of excessive processed foods, sugary snacks, or unhealthy fats.

4. Mindful Eating:

Keep practicing mindful eating to maintain a healthy relationship with food. Pay attention to portion sizes and eat with awareness.

5. Regular Exercise:

Continue with your regular exercise routine. Adjust the intensity and type of exercise as needed, but make sure physical activity remains a consistent part of your life.

6. Stay Hydrated:

Maintain proper hydration by drinking an adequate amount of water each day. Hydration is essential for overall health and metabolic function.

7. Manage Stress:

Continue to manage stress through techniques such as meditation, yoga, or deep breathing exercises. High stress levels can negatively impact your metabolic health.

8. Sleep:

Prioritize quality sleep, aiming for 7-9 hours each night. Sleep plays a significant role in metabolic health and overall well-being.

9. Celebrate Success:

Celebrate your achievements and milestones. Acknowledge your progress and use these celebrations as motivation to stay on track.

10. Be Adaptable:

Be open to making adjustments as needed. Life is dynamic, and there may be periods when you need to adapt your routines. Don't view these changes as setbacks but as part of the journey.

11. Support System:

Stay connected with your support system, whether it's friends, family, or a community of like-minded individuals. They can offer motivation and encouragement.

12. Learn Continuously:

Keep learning about nutrition and health. Staying informed about new developments can help you make informed choices.

13. Periodic Assessments:

Periodically assess your metabolic health through check-ups and evaluations. Regular monitoring can help you catch any potential issues early.

14. Set New Goals:

Consider setting new health and fitness goals to keep your journey exciting and challenging. Having new objectives can maintain your motivation.

15. Long-Term Perspective:

Remember that metabolic health is a lifelong commitment. Continue to focus on well-being and consider it as a permanent aspect of your life.

16. Help Others:

Share your knowledge and experiences with others who may be on a similar journey. Providing support and guidance to others can be rewarding and help reinforce your own commitment.

By following these post-metabolic reset guidelines, you can continue to enjoy the benefits of improved metabolic health and overall well-being. The key is to maintain your healthy habits, stay adaptable, and prioritize your long-term health and vitality.

Incorporating Variety into Your Diet

Incorporating variety into your diet is essential for several reasons, including providing a wide range of nutrients, preventing dietary boredom, and maintaining a healthy relationship with food. Here are tips for introducing variety into your diet:

1. Explore Different Food Groups:

Make it a point to include foods from all food groups, such as fruits, vegetables, whole grains, lean proteins, and healthy fats, in your meals. Each group provides unique nutrients and flavors.

2. Seasonal Eating:

Embrace seasonal produce. Fruits and vegetables that are in season tend to be fresher, tastier, and more affordable. Plus, they can add variety to your diet throughout the year.

3. Try New Recipes:

Experiment with new recipes and cooking techniques. There are countless cuisines and dishes to explore, each with its unique set of ingredients and flavors.

4. Mix Protein Sources:

Diversify your sources of protein. Include plant-based options like beans, lentils, and tofu in addition to animal proteins like poultry, fish, and lean meats.

5. Colorful Plates:

Aim to have a colorful plate. Different colors in your meals often indicate a variety of nutrients. A colorful salad, for example, can include greens, red peppers, purple onions, and yellow tomatoes.

6. Whole Grains Variety:

Choose a variety of whole grains, such as quinoa, brown rice, whole wheat pasta, and oats. They not only add diversity but also provide essential nutrients and fiber.

7. Experiment with Spices and Herbs:

Enhance your dishes with various spices and herbs. These can completely transform the flavor of your meals. Explore international cuisines for inspiration.

8. Meal Planning:

Plan your meals to ensure you incorporate a mix of foods. Creating a weekly meal plan can help you organize your menu and include diverse options.

9. Seasonal Fruits and Vegetables:

Seasonal fruits and vegetables are often more affordable and flavorful. They can also add variety to your meals and snacks.

10. Food Swaps:

Make simple swaps to diversify your diet. For example, replace regular pasta with whole wheat pasta or white rice with quinoa.

11. Breakfast Variations:

Experiment with different breakfast options. Instead of the same cereal every day, try oatmeal, yogurt with fruits, smoothies, or scrambled eggs.

12. Snack Smart:

Choose a range of healthy snacks, such as nuts, seeds, yogurt, hummus with veggies, or fresh fruit. This can break the monotony of snacking.

13. Cultural Exploration:

Explore the foods of different cultures. Trying dishes from around the world can be a fun way to incorporate variety into your diet.

14. Listen to Cravings:

Sometimes, your body may be craving specific nutrients or flavors. Pay attention to your cravings and incorporate healthier versions of what you desire.

15. Regularly Update Your Grocery List:

Review and update your grocery list regularly. This can prompt you to try new foods or ingredients.

16. Share Meals:

Share meals with friends and family who may have different culinary traditions and preferences. It's a great way to explore different cuisines.

Remember that variety doesn't mean sacrificing your dietary goals. You can maintain a balanced and nutritious diet while enjoying a wide range of foods. Regularly incorporating variety into your diet not only keeps your meals interesting but also supports your overall health and metabolic well-being.

CHAPTER TWELVE

BEYOND WEIGHT LOSS

Improving Energy Levels

Improving your energy levels is a common goal of metabolic resets and is essential for overall well-being. Here are some strategies to boost and sustain your energy throughout the day:

Balanced Diet:

Consume a balanced diet that includes a mix of macronutrients (carbohydrates, proteins, and healthy fats) and micronutrients (vitamins and minerals). Opt for whole foods like fruits, vegetables, lean proteins, and whole grains.

Regular Meals:

Eat regular, balanced meals and snacks. Skipping meals can lead to energy crashes. Aim for three meals and two to three snacks a day to maintain stable blood sugar levels.

Stay Hydrated:

Dehydration can lead to fatigue. Ensure you're drinking enough water throughout the day. Herbal teas and infused water can also contribute to hydration.

Control Portion Sizes:

Overeating can make you feel sluggish. Practice portion control to avoid overloading your digestive system.

Complex Carbohydrates:

Include complex carbohydrates like whole grains, legumes, and starchy vegetables in your meals. These provide sustained energy and prevent blood sugar spikes and crashes.

Protein Intake:

Protein-rich foods like lean meats, dairy, and plant-based sources (e.g., beans, tofu) help maintain muscle mass and provide lasting energy.

Healthy Fats:

Include sources of healthy fats such as avocados, nuts, and olive oil in your diet. They can provide a slow and steady release of energy.

Limit Added Sugars:

Excessive sugar intake can lead to energy fluctuations. Minimize added sugars and opt for natural sources of sweetness like fruits.

Fiber-Rich Foods:

Foods high in fiber, such as fruits, vegetables, and whole grains, help regulate blood sugar and keep you feeling full and energized.

Balanced Snacks:

Choose balanced snacks that combine carbohydrates, protein, and healthy fats. For example, Greek yogurt with berries and a sprinkle of almonds.

Regular Exercise:

Physical activity, even a brisk walk, can boost energy levels. Aim for at least 150 minutes of moderate exercise per week.

Manage Stress:

High stress levels can lead to fatigue. Practice stress management techniques like deep breathing, meditation, or yoga to improve your energy and mood.

Adequate Sleep:

Ensure you get enough quality sleep. Adults generally need 7-9 hours of sleep per night. A good sleep routine contributes significantly to energy levels.

Limit Caffeine and Alcohol:

While moderate caffeine can provide a temporary energy boost, excessive caffeine or alcohol consumption can disrupt sleep and lead to energy crashes.

Regular Mealtimes:

Try to eat meals at consistent times each day. Regular meal patterns can help regulate your body's internal clock and improve energy levels.

Stay Active:

Even when you're not exercising, stay active throughout the day. Take short breaks to stretch and move around, especially if you have a sedentary job.

Hydrotherapy:

Alternating between hot and cold showers or using cold water splashes can help invigorate and boost energy.

Breathe Deeply:

Take deep, slow breaths when you're feeling fatigued. Deep breathing can oxygenate your body and increase alertness.

Set Realistic Goals:

Manage your expectations and set realistic goals to reduce stress and prevent burnout.

Stay Positive:

Maintain a positive outlook and focus on activities and people that energize you.

Improving and maintaining your energy levels is a multifaceted endeavor. Experiment with these strategies to find what works best for you and consider consulting a healthcare professional or registered dietitian for personalized guidance.

Supporting Overall Wellness

Supporting overall wellness is a holistic approach that encompasses physical, mental, and emotional well-being. Here are some strategies to help you achieve and maintain wellness in all aspects of your life:

1. Balanced Nutrition:

Prioritize a balanced diet rich in whole foods, including fruits, vegetables, lean proteins, whole grains, and healthy fats. Avoid excessive processed foods, added sugars, and unhealthy fats.

2. Regular Exercise:

Incorporate physical activity into your daily routine. Aim for a mix of cardiovascular exercise, strength training, and flexibility exercises to improve overall fitness.

3. Hydration:

Stay adequately hydrated by drinking water throughout the day. Water is essential for all bodily functions and overall well-being.

4. Quality Sleep:

Prioritize quality sleep by establishing a consistent sleep schedule and creating a comfortable sleep environment. Aim for 7-9 hours of sleep per night.

5. Stress Management:

Practice stress management techniques such as deep breathing, meditation, yoga, or mindfulness to reduce stress and promote emotional well-being.

6. Mental Health Support:

Seek support when needed. Talk to a mental health professional if you're experiencing anxiety, depression, or other emotional challenges. It's essential to address mental health as part of overall wellness.

7. Social Connections:

Cultivate meaningful relationships with friends and family. Social connections are vital for emotional and mental well-being.

8. Purpose and Meaning:

Identify your values and goals, and strive to find purpose and meaning in your daily activities. Having a sense of purpose can boost overall wellness.

9. Time Management:

Manage your time effectively to reduce stress and find a balance between work, leisure, and self-care.

10. Regular Check-Ups:

Schedule regular check-ups with your healthcare provider to monitor your physical health. Early detection of health issues is crucial for overall wellness.

11. Self-Care:

Dedicate time to self-care activities that you enjoy. Whether it's reading, taking a bath, or pursuing a hobby, self-care is essential for mental and emotional well-being.

12. Holistic Wellness:

Take a holistic approach to wellness by considering the mind-body connection. Physical health, mental health, and emotional health are interconnected and affect overall wellness.

13. Goal Setting:

Set and work toward personal and professional goals. Having objectives can provide a sense of purpose and direction in life.

14. Environmental Wellness:

Create a clean and organized living space that promotes well-being. A clutter-free environment can reduce stress and promote mental clarity.

15. Spiritual Wellness:

Explore your spirituality and engage in practices that align with your beliefs. This can provide a sense of inner peace and fulfillment.

16. Financial Wellness:

Manage your finances responsibly to reduce financial stress. Create a budget, save, and plan for the future.

17. Lifelong Learning:

Continue to learn and grow throughout your life. Acquiring new skills and knowledge can contribute to overall wellness.

18. Gratitude and Positivity:

Cultivate a mindset of gratitude and positivity. Focus on the good in your life and practice gratitude daily.

19. Giving Back:

Engage in acts of kindness and giving back to your community. Volunteering and helping others can enhance your overall sense of well-being.

20. Balance and Adaptability:

Maintain a balanced and adaptable approach to wellness. Life is dynamic, and your needs may change over time. Be open to adjusting your wellness strategies.

Remember that wellness is a lifelong journey, and it's essential to continually assess and adapt your approach to meet your changing needs. Prioritize self-care, stay attuned to your physical and emotional health, and seek support and guidance as needed to achieve overall wellness.

CONCLUSION

Your Future with A Revitalized Metabolism

In conclusion, a revitalized metabolism can significantly impact your future, enhancing your overall health, energy levels, and well-being. By undertaking a metabolic reset, you're making an investment in yourself that can yield numerous benefits for years to come. As you look toward the future with a healthier metabolism, consider the following key points:

1. **Lifelong Well-Being:** A metabolic reset isn't just a temporary fix; it's a commitment to lifelong well-being. By adopting sustainable habits and making positive changes, you're setting yourself up for a healthier, more energetic, and fulfilling life.

2. **Preventative Health:** A revitalized metabolism reduces the risk of various chronic diseases, including diabetes, heart disease, and obesity. It's an investment in your long-term health and quality of life.

3. **Improved Energy:** With a healthier metabolism, you'll enjoy increased energy levels and vitality. This can positively impact your daily activities and help you pursue your passions and goals with enthusiasm.

4. **Mental Clarity:** Better metabolic health can lead to improved cognitive function, helping you think more clearly,

concentrate better, and maintain mental sharpness as you age.

5. **Emotional Well-Being:** A metabolic reset can also have a positive impact on your emotional well-being. It can help reduce stress, anxiety, and depression, fostering a more balanced and content outlook on life.

6. **Physical Fitness:** A revitalized metabolism supports your physical fitness and athletic performance. Whether you're an athlete or someone who enjoys regular physical activity, a healthier metabolism can help you excel.

7. **Longevity:** By focusing on your metabolic health, you're taking steps to extend your lifespan and enhance your quality of life as you age.

8. **Positive Habits:** The habits you establish during a metabolic reset become a part of your daily routine. These habits contribute to a healthier lifestyle that can benefit you for years to come.

9. **Personal Growth:** Improved well-being often fosters personal growth. You'll have the energy, health, and mindset to pursue new challenges and explore new opportunities.

10. **Inspirational Impact:** Your journey toward better metabolic health can serve as an inspiration to those around

you. Your commitment to well-being can positively influence friends and family to make similar changes.

As you embark on or continue your metabolic reset journey, remember that it's a personal and unique path. What works for one person may not be suitable for another. Consult with healthcare professionals or registered dietitians to tailor your approach to your individual needs and goals.

Your future with a revitalized metabolism is one filled with health, vitality, and endless possibilities. Embrace the journey, stay committed to your well-being, and look forward to a brighter, healthier, and more fulfilling future.

Printed in Great Britain
by Amazon